Olaf Evjenth & Jern Hamberg

MUSCLE STRETCHING IN MANUAL THERAPY

A Clinical Manual

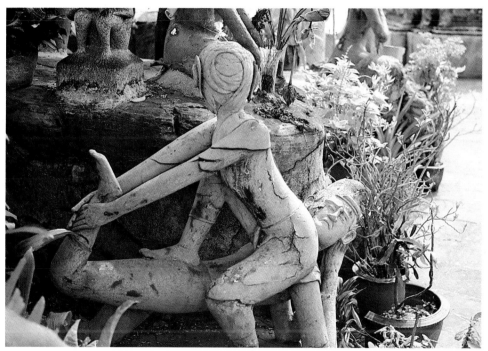

Muscle stretching 2000 years ago. Statue from Bangkok.

Volume I The Extremities

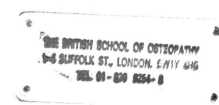

ALFTA REHAB

MUSCLE STRETCHING IN MANUAL THERAPY, A CLINICAL MANUAL, TWO VOLUMES

OLAF EVJENTH, M.S.
LECTURER IN MANUAL THERAPY,
HANS & OLAF INSTITUTE
OSLO, NORWAY

AND

JERN HAMBERG, M.D.
DIRECTOR,
ALFTA REHABILITATION CENTER
ALFTA, SWEDEN

ALFTA REHAB FØRLAG
Box 93
S-822 00 Alfta
Sweden

Edited by M. Michael Brady
Photos by Bjørn Hamberg
Drawings by Elna Jonsson

Production by Scand Book AB Sweden
Printed by New Intherlitho Spa, Milan, Italy 1985.

ISBN 91-85934-02-X

Today, one patient in four seeking medical aid does so solely with a locomotor system complaint. Many of the remaining three-quarters of all patients seeking medical aid primarily for other reasons also complain of stiffness, aches, and painful movement. The muscular-skeletal disorders of patients in these two categories comprise the greatest single cause of sick leave. The persons affected dominate the group of those who retire early on disability pensions. The socio-economic problems resulting from muscular-skeletal disorders are undoubtedly greater and more widespread than indicated by any single statistic.

Years of research and experience in studying and treating locomotor system maladies have clearly proven the effectiveness of treatment through relaxation and stretching of shortened muscles and other related structures. The techniques involved are basically therapeutic, but they may also be applied in preventative exercise at all levels of physical training programs, for persons of all ages.

Our research has been pragmatically oriented towards attaining results for a greater number of patients over longer periods of time. Hence we have not conducted double-blind tests, but instead have allowed our patients to function as their own controls. Prolonged dysfunction, which diminishes dramatically after relaxation and stretching treatment, is more than ample proof of treatment effectiveness, both for the therapist and for the patients involved.

This book is a compendium of therapeutic techniques that we have used to successfully treat patients with reduced mobility caused by shortened structures. Treatments for the extremities and their associated joints are covered in **Volume I**. Treatments for the spine and the temporo-mandibular joint are covered in **Volume II**. Although the temporo-mandibular joint is anatomically removed from the spine, it is therapeutically recognized as being closely connected to the cervical spine and therefore is included in **Volume II**. Each of the two Volumes is arranged to be used as an independent clinical reference.

In this **Volume I**:

The general principles of manual therapy are outlined in **Part 1**, along with a guide to the organization of the therapy techniques. The therapy techniques are fully described in **Part 2** and **Part 3**, one to a page. Each description consists of a drawing showing the muscles involved, two photos showing the starting and final positions of the technique, and an explicit text giving positions, grips and procedures.

The Movement Restriction Tables and Index of Muscles of **Part 4** list the muscles which may restrict movement and reference them to pages.

The two volumes of this book are intended primarily to be used as ready-reference clinical manuals and as texts on muscle stretching in manual therapy. However, we hope that they will also provide physiotherapists and medical doctors with a fresh, comprehensive approach to the entire subject of muscle stretching in manual therapy. Our underlying goal has been to contribute to improving the quality of the treatment of muscular-skeletal disorders, both for patients and for therapists. We will be pleased if the users of this manual find it useful in realizing that goal.

Oslo, Norway and Alfta, Sweden
August 1984
Olaf Evjenth and Jern Hamberg

CONTENTS

PART 1

GENERAL PRINCIPLES OF RELAXATION AND STRETCHING OF MUSCLES AND OTHER STRUCTURES

1. GENERAL PRINCIPLES OF RELAXATION AND STRETCHING OF MUSCLES AND OTHER STRUCTURES

1.1. INTRODUCTION

Humans have always been physically active for reasons other than pure necessity. Nonessential activities, which now classify physiologically as exercise or stretching, evolved for reasons long forgotten or never recorded. Although dance and ritual were obvious progenitors, non-productive physical activity undoubtedly had utilitarian origins: Its early practitioners felt better after stretching. Historical confirmation of the origins of exercise and stretching is lacking. But there's ample evidence that stretching, such as that depicted by the 2000 year old statue shown in the frontispiece of this book, has been practiced since the dawn of history.

Stretching now divides into *therapeutic stretching*, the topic of this Manual and *self-stretching*, as used in exercise, athletic training, dance, and certain ritual exercises. The two categories of stretching may supplement each other. For instance, therapists may teach their patients self-stretching to speed recovery, and sports teams may employ therapists to treat athletes. Yet there is good reason to differentiate. Controlled, proper stretching is beneficial. But uncontrolled stretching of muscles and other structures may damage, such as through causing instability or pathological hypermobility. In most such cases, self-stretching is involved.

Unwary athletes and other persons exercising often self-stretch with great force at long lever arms, which easily injures. Some competitive athletic events, such as gymnastics in general and women's gymnastics in particular, require extreme movement and therefore frequently injure participants. Other extreme activities, such as group exercises to music ("jazzexercise" and "aerobic dance" are two) also pose high hazard of stretching damage. Some exercises are faulted, but lack of knowledge is the leading underlying cause of self-stretching damage. Most people know little of the normal ranges of movement of the joints of their bodies. The result is that when they stretch, normal structures are often overstretched, while shortened structures are seldom adequately stretched.

An understanding of why, when and how muscles or other structures should be stretched is prerequisite to stretching to benefit rather than degrade body function. The role of the therapist in stretching is then not just to understand and treat, but also to guide and teach patients self-stretching (see references 6 and 7).

1.2. INDICATIONS

Every patient with symptoms involving the locomotor system, particularly symptoms of pain and/or constrained movement, should be examined to assess joint and muscle function. If examination shows joint play to be normal, but reveals shortened muscles or muscle spasm, then treatment by stretching is indicated. With a view towards preventive medicine, all younger children should be examined and, if necessary, treated for any disturbed muscle function before symptoms appear.

1.3. CONTRAINDICATIONS

Any dysfunction and/or pain of suspected pathological origin contraindicates manual therapy. Affected patients should be advised to seek medical diagnosis, and return to therapy if their doctors negate the suspected pathology and recommend return.

1.4. GUIDELINES FOR THE THERAPIST

The only reliable way to become proficient in detecting and treating muscle dysfunction is through experience gained by *thoroughly examining every patient*. Unfortunately there are no exact rules for examination. Normal ranges of movement referenced in texts, though typical of large populations, are seldom directly applicable in individual cases and therefore do not always indicate if muscles and/or other structures need stretching. So patient examinations should start with *preliminary biomechanical analyses*.

If the preliminary analysis identifies shortened muscles, then a provisional trial treatment is performed. If the provisional treatment reduces pain and improves the affected movement pattern, the preliminary analysis is confirmed, and treatment may proceed. The restoration of the muscles' *normal pattern of movement*, with *freedom from pain*, is the *only real measure* by which the treatment may be judged to have been successful. With experience, examiners can detect particular shortened muscles that constrain movement in their surrounding structures. Sometimes movement patterns and/or ranges of movements cannot be fully restored because of irreversible damage or changes in locomotive structures. Nonetheless, stretching can still be valuable in treatment.

The starting positions, Fig. a, of the techniques of Part 3, correspond to positions imposed by shortening, while the final positions, Fig. b, correspond to extent of maximum range of movement.

1.5. DYSFUNCTION

1.5.1. Causes and Mechanisms

When functioning normally, a muscle has optimum circulation and innervation, is able to move freely, is unimpaired in contracting and relaxing, and has normal elasticity and strength. All movements should be free of pain. Muscle function may depart from this norm in many ways, primarily because muscles are among the most susceptible of body structures. They must continually readjust to their use, disuse, or misuse. Muscle shortening frequently results. Stiff or shortened muscles are often activated in movements in which they otherwise would not take part. This overuse in turn leads to injury and/or to excess inhibition of their antagonists. In general, the shorter the muscle, the more it may inhibit its antagonists. Therefore, stimulating and strengthening a muscle's antagonists always aids treatment. However, note that *the shortened muscle being treated should always be stretched before its antagonists are strengthened.*

Shortened muscles may cause pain from the periosteum, tendons, or muscle belly, including referred pain to other structures or segments. In a synergistic group, no one muscle should be shorter than the others of the group. A stiff, shortened muscle will be subjected to greater stress when contracted suddenly and forcefully, thus damaging itself and/or its associated tendon. This can be prevented by stretching the relevant muscle or muscle group.

Normal range of movement is determined by several structures: skin, subcutaneous tissue, muscles, ligaments, joint capsules, joint surfaces, and intraarticular structures. Changes in any of these structures alter ranges of movement. Conditions such as septic or aseptic inflammations may cause restricted movements when acute, and pathological instability when chronic. The structures most affected are the fascia, joint capsules, ligaments, and joint cartilages. An example is the development of *ankylosing spondylarthritis* (Morbus Bechterew). An initial instability becomes hypomobility through degenerative change. Subsequent development may further restrict movement ranges, and occasionally lead to ankylosis. If a reduced range of movement is caused by shortened muscles, then treatment by stretching increases and may restore the range of movement to normal.

1.5.2. Symptoms

Dysfunction due to shortened structures can be detected by observing one or more of the following changes it may cause:
1. Pattern of movement,
2. Volume and swelling and/or distention of a muscle,
3. Elasticity of a muscle,
4. Range of movement at a joint,
5. Joint play (section **1.6.3**, p. 9),
6. Quality of the passive stop, end feel (section 1.6.3, p. 9); *most important.*

In addition to these indicators, a patient may experience fatigue, pain radiating to other muscles and structures, and a feeling of stiffness in the shortened muscle(s). Shortened muscles may also irritate and damage peripheral nerves and blood vessels; examples include sports injuries, and the scalenus, the supinator, the pronator and piriformis syndromes. Poor physical condition, inadequate coordination, or unaccustomed movement often cause altered circulation and faulty muscle movement patterns. According to Vladimir Janda(1), this leads to constant *micro-traumata*, which, in turn, subsequently effects alterations in patterns of movement with chronic muscle spasm, contractures and pain. In an advanced case, joint function is altered and degenerative changes at the joints result. Stretching of the relevant muscle(s) is one way of *preventing* this chain of events.

1.6. MANUAL THERAPY METHODS

1.6.1. The Basics of Stretching

All therapy techniques including stretching should be based on thorough examination. Stretching techniques differ primarily by the type and degree of patient involvement in procedures administered by the therapist. Common to all procedures is a basic, safest sequence of events based on the principle that a muscle is most relaxed and therefore may be maximally stretched immediately after an isometric contraction. According to Sherrington(2), the stronger the contraction (without pain), the greater the subsequent relaxation.

So all procedures start with a static *contraction* of the shortened muscle(s). Then the muscles are relaxed, which makes them more easily stretched for a period of a fraction of a second up to 10 or 12 seconds in pathological cases. During this period, the muscles can be safely stretched. Often patients cannot contract from an extreme position, so treatment procedure cannot begin there. In these cases, it is best to move back to a position in the range of movement where the patient can easily contract, and begin the procedure there.

Muscles are most amenable to stretching when they are *warmed up* in the physiological sense, by preliminary exercise rather than by the application of passive, external heat. Thus all treatment should start with some form of warmup. The best and most specific warmup exercise is contraction against resistance. The stronger the contraction, the greater the warmup effect.

Unwanted external stimuli, such as noise or discomfort, can impair treatment, particularly treatments requiring combined efforts of patient and therapist. So the patient should always be made as comfortable as possible. The treatment surroundings should be quiet, and other distracting influences should be eliminated whenever possible.

1.6.2. Therapy Procedures

In all therapy procedures, the therapist works to counteract some restriction of movement about a joint. Three different therapeutic approaches are possible, depending on whether the patient is completely passive, participates by offering resistance, or participates both by offering resistance and by working with the therapist.

1. Patient passive: This technique is used in treating more serious contractures to produce lasting lengthening of shortened tissue. The patient relaxes while the therapist moves the joint further in the direction of restriction, and then holds the extreme position as long as necessary, even up to two minutes or more, to lengthen the shortened structures.

2. Patient resists: In this gentle technique, the therapist applies moderate force to move a joint as far as possible in the direction of restriction. The shortened structures then press the joint surfaces together. Then the therapist applies traction at the joint, and thus tries to separate the joint surfaces as the patient resists. Thereafter, the patient relaxes and the therapist maintains traction as long as necessary, until the joint surfaces are felt to separate. The procedure is repeated until movement is appreciably improved.

3. Patient resists and aids: This is the *recommended technique* of this Manual. It starts as does the "Patient resists" technique above, but differs thereafter. First, the therapist moves a joint as far as possible in the direction of restriction. Then the therapist holds the position and asks the patient to isometrically resist it. Patient and therapist should resist each other equally, with the patient contracting one or all of the muscles which are to be stretched; this ensures negligible joint movement. The patient then relaxes while the therapist moves the joint further in the direction of restriction. The process is repeated until improvement is attained. In some cases when the therapist moves a joint, the patient either feels pain or fears pain to an extent that blocks relaxation. The therapist can then apply traction and aid or even offer slight resistance as the patient actively moves the joint in the direction of restriction. Thus the patient controls movement and therefore can relax. In all cases, the therapist holds the extreme position as long as necessary, even up to two minutes or more, to lengthen the shortened structures.

1.6.3. Character of Joint Movement

In treating joints, the therapist should continually assess the quality and quantity of joint movement and the manner in which movement stops. These evaluations then guide the course of further therapy. For instance, some joint movement abnormalities may contraindicate stretching therapy.

1. *Joint Play*

Joint play is the gliding and/or separation of joint surfaces without angular movement about a joint. All joints have a characteristic joint play, with which the therapist should be familiar. Normally joint play is greatest in the maximally loose-packed position and diminishes to minima at the extremes of the joint range of movement. The therapist must always examine a joint for joint play before using any of the treatment procedures described above. If joint play is less than normal, it must be restored to normal before other therapy is begun or continued.

2. *End Feel*

The therapist must be able to sense the extremes of the various possible ranges of movements about body joints, that is, the points at which passive movement stops (3,4). **End feel** is the sensation imparted to the therapist at these points. There are several different types of end feel; the therapist must be able to differentiate between them:

Normal end feel may be *soft, firm or hard*:

Soft: Soft tissue approximation and/or stretching, such as knee or elbow flexion with normally-developed muscles.

Firm: Capsule and/or ligament stretching, such as medial rotation of the humerus or femur.

Hard: Bone-to-bone stop, such as elbow extension.

Abnormal end feel: Abnormalities may produce varying end feels; six are differentiated:

Less-elastic: Such as due to scar tissue or shortened connective tissue.

More-elastic: Such as due to increased muscle tonus, shortened muscles.

Springy block: Internal derangement where the rebound is seen and felt, such as due to torn meniscus.

"Empty": The patient feels severe pain, such as due to acute bursitis, extraarticular abscess or neoplasm, and will not permit the movement to go further; no physical stop felt by the therapist.

Premature: Occurs *before* normal stop, such as in rheumatoid arthritis or osteoarthrosis, or contracted ligaments or capsules.

Extended: Occurs *after* normal stop, such as in cases of instability or hypermobility.

1.7. RECOMMENDED THERAPY PROCEDURE

The therapy techniques of Section 3 involve the patient resisting and aiding, the third of the three approaches to procedure described in **1.6.2**, p. 9. In these techniques:

* The therapist moves a patient's joint(s), in the direction of restriction, to positions progressively approaching, but never exceeding the normal range of joint motion, as determined by end feel.

* The patient actively participates in the treatment procedure, alternately resisting or aiding motion as directed by the therapist.

* Successive sequences of isometric contraction, relaxation and stretching are used to attain the desired improvement in joint movement range, followed by stimulation of the antagonists. Descriptions of these treatment phases follow.

1.7.1. Isometric Contraction

First, the therapist moves the joint(s) to a position in the line of movement to less than that which might cause pain. It may be possible to start in a position with the shortened structures relatively stretched. However, it is often necessary to start in a position where the patient can easily resist the movement.

Then, in this position, the patient is instructed to resist movement by isometrically contracting the shortened muscle(s). In this **phase, the therapist and the patient apply forces that counterbalance so there is no movement in the joint itself.** The therapist's grip and resistance applied must be comfortable, painless, and secure for the patient.

If isometric contraction causes the patient no pain, the therapist can readily and rapidly tire the muscle(s) involved by applying sufficient resistance (relative to the contracting muscular force) for a few seconds or longer. If the isometric contraction is painful for the patient, then the therapist should decrease resistance and increase the period of force counterbalance, up to 10 to 30 seconds.

1.7.2. Relaxation

When the therapist feels that the patient has sufficiently contracted the shortened muscle(s), the patient is instructed to relax. As the patient relaxes, the therapist releases resistance accordingly, so as not to cause pain or unwanted movement(s).

1.7.3. Stretching to Counteract and Reduce Restriction

After the preceding isometric contraction and relaxation, movement may be improved in four ways:

1. The therapist moves the joint in the direction of restriction.
2. If this movement is painful or if the patient fears pain, then the therapist may be more passive and let the patient actively move at the joint.
3. Pain experienced often may be lessened considerably if the therapist applies gentle traction while the patient actively moves at the joint.
4. Sometimes pain may be further reduced if, in addition to applying gentle traction, the therapist also simultaneously either:
   a) aids the patient's movement at the joint, or
   b) provides *gentle resistance* while the patient moves at the joint.

Once an initial new position is attained, the sequence of contraction, relaxation and stretching is successively repeated to progressively attain the desired improvement in movement range. Thereafter, the antagonist(s) should be stimulated.

1.7.4. Stimulation of Antagonists

The antagonists to the muscle(s) treated always should be stimulated immediately after the sequence of treatment to increase movement in the direction of restriction.

To stimulate the antagonists, the therapist reverses the direction of force or resistance applied, and counteracts movement. To reverse the direction of force applied, the therapist may either retain grip or change grip, depending on the treatment technique involved. Once the therapist is prepared to apply a reverse force, the patient is asked to move in the direction just stretched in the treatment, and the therapist opposes that movement to evaluate the ability and the force with which the antagonists contract.

Inhibition of antagonists can be reduced through vigorous stimulation, such as rapid vibrating movements, pinching and shaking/stretching muscles, slapping the skin, or traction or compression (approximation) of the joint(s).

Restricted joint mobility or pain may inhibit and thus lead to weakening of the antagonists. Therefore it may be necessary to strengthen these muscles throughout their full range of movement. The muscles should be able to control movement through the full range and should also be able to lock the joint in any position in that range. Stimulation of the antagonists is always a vital part of successful treatment.

Neurological dysfunction may block or mask a patient's perception of stimuli. In these cases, stimulation must be confined to localized areas. For instance, in stimulating the finger flexor muscles (antagonists to the finger extensors), the therapist should apply pressure only to the volar sides of the fingers.

1.7.5. Stretching of Other Structures

Whenever successive contraction and relaxation treatments fail to increase movement at a joint, the joint should be reexamined to ascertain if the restriction is caused by structures other than muscle(s), such as by ligaments or joint capsules. If joint play is noticably diminished or absent, it may be restored using joint mobilization techniques, such as those described by Kaltenborn(3) and Stoddard(5). However, if joint glide is normal but movement is restricted, the following procedure may be used. The therapist stretches the shortened structures by applying an *optimal intensity* force. *Intensity* is the combination of force magnitude and duration of application, with duration being the more important in stretching. *Optimal* means as small as possible, yet adequate for results: a small force for a few seconds to two minutes or more.

The patient should feel the stretching, possibly even as pain, though not to the point of serious discomfort. **Elsewhere the treatment should cause no pain.** If the procedure produces no improvement, the force applied may have been of insufficient intensity. If so, stretching should be repeated at greater intensity, preferably for longer periods of time, and then if necessary, with greater force.

Physiotherapists or doctors may administer these therapeutic stretching techniques. However, therapy is more effective if it is supplemented by more frequent self stretching, preferably daily or several times a day. Therefore, patients should be taught self stretching (6,7). In general, the more frequent the stretching, the more moderate the intensity. Less frequent stretching, such as that done every other day, may be at greater intensity.

1.8   TECHNIQUES – PARTS 2 AND 3

1.8.1   Caveat

In all treatments, the therapist should strive to avoid compression at joints if possible, and, if not, to minimize it as much as treatment permits. Compression may hinder desired movements at articulations, can stress nerve tissue, or otherwise damage joints or their immediate structures. Therefore, traction should be used in all procedures as a means of counteracting any compression which may arise as a result of the movement the therapist induces.

1.8.2   Key to Therapy Techniques

Detailed descriptions of the techniques used to stretch restricting structures are arranged in eight sections in Parts 2 and 3: shoulder, elbow, wrist, fingers, hip, knee, ankle, toes.

Each of these sections starts with a Therapy Guide containing two tables. The first table lists the possible restrictions at the joint, the muscles which may cause each of the restrictions, and the therapies for those muscles, indexed by number and page.

Alternative therapies for any particular restriction are indicated by suffix letters. For instance, there are two techniques for the pectoralis major, abdominal part listed in section 2.2.1:

2.2.1.A

Section 2 on the shoulder

Subsection 2.2 on restricted flexion

Therapies 2.2.1 for Technique A, the pectoralis major, bilateral stretching abdominal part

For uniformity, all technique descriptions are similar. In all cases where either the right or left joint may be treated, the right is shown and discussed. The therapist then reads right for left and vice versa in the equivalent therapy on the patient's left.

Each therapy is illustrated with a muscle drawing and starting and final position photos. X in illustrations indicates points of stabilization by hands, belts etc. Arrows in illustrations indicate directions of stretching movements and also patient movement in the antagonist muscle stimulation phase. P in texts denotes the patient, T the therapist.

All instructions are for you, the Therapist, and are divided into four parts: Starting Position, Grip, Procedure and Stimulation of Antagonists. When needed, Notes clarify or supplement these four parts.

The Starting Position instructions consist of short statements on how to arrange the patient and yourself to start treatment. They may easily be remembered if you view them as brief descriptions of a scene, or as notes you might take upon first seeing the technique performed by another therapists.

The other three instructions, Grip, Procedure and Stimulation of Antagonists are direct instructions on how to perform the treatment.

Instructions for the patient also require monitoring by the therapist. For instance, some Procedure instructions require the patient to keep his/her chin tucked in during treatment. You should then ask the patient to tuck his/her chin in while preparing for treatment, and you also must continually watch the patient during treatment to be sure that the tuck is maintained.

Note that most stretching should be performed gradually and fully, so the origin and insertion of the muscles are moved as far apart as possible, approaching but not going beyond the normal range of movement.

As in anatomy texts, the descriptions of muscle action of this Manual assume starting in the anatomical position. However, muscle action may change at an extreme joint position, sometimes to the opposite of that described. For instance, when starting from the anatomical position, the adductors of the hip flex at the hip joint, yet they act as extensors at full hip flexion. This is why full range of movement sometimes can be attained only by stretching from different starting positions. Complete tables of muscles involved in restricting various movements are given in Part 4.

1.8.4   Terminology

Standard anatomic terminology is used throughout this Manual. However, whenever two or more synonymous anatomical terms are in accepted current use, the terms most pertinent to the physiotherapy situation are used.

Because manual therapy is concerned with joints and muscles and related structures, all descriptions of therapy procedures and of muscle actions are in terms of joint movements. For instance, the action of the biceps brachii muscle of the upper arm is described as "flexes at the elbow," while a medical anatomy text author might prefer "flexes arm and forearm."

In summary, the terminology of this Manual may be viewed as chosen to suit an active situation, in which the therapist promotes, directs, or elicits motion, as opposed to some surgical or medical choices of terms, which may be viewed as more passive, intended primarily for identification or description.

1.8.5   Using the Ready Reference Features

The ready reference features of this Manual can best be explained by example. Assume an adult female patient, who complains that she is unable to manipulate the strap clasp of her brassiere because she cannot reach her mid back with her right hand. The restricted movements involve various degrees of extension, adduction and medial rotation at the shoulder. First, Section 2 on the shoulder is found either by page number from the Contents or by flipping through the pages to find The Shoulder at the top of the pages involved. Table 2-1 lists the restricted movement under subsection 2.8, with eight muscles which may cause restriction and the corresponding therapies, listed by number and page number. All primary and secondary restricting muscles are listeed in Table 10-1 of the Muscle Restriction Tables on page 165.

1.9. REFERENCES

1. Janda, Vladimir, "Die Bedeutung der muskulären Fehlhaltung als pathogenetischer Faktor vertebrangener Störungen," **Arch. physikal. Therapie, 20** (1968), 113-116.

2. Sherrington, C.S., "On plastic tonus and proprioceptive reflexes," **Quart. J. Exp. Physiol., 2** (1909), 109-156.

3. Kaltenborn, Freddy M., **Manual Therapy for the Extremity Joints**, Oslo, Olaf Norlis Bokhandel, 1980.

4. Cyriax, James, **Textbook of Orthopedic Medicine**, London, Hutchinson, 1969.

5. Stoddard, Alan, **Manual of Osteopathic Technique**, London, Hutchinson, 1980.

6. Gunnari, Hans, and Evjenth, Olaf, **Sequence Exercise**, Oslo, Dreyers Forlag, Norwegian edition 1983, English edition 1984 (Chapter 7 on self-stretching)

7. Evjenth, Olaf, and Hamberg, Jern, **Self Stretching**, in press.

PART 2

THERAPY TECHNIQUES FOR THE UPPER EXTREMITY

2 THE SHOULDER

3 THE ELBOW

4 THE WRIST

5 THE FINGERS

2 THE SHOULDER

2.1 THERAPY GUIDE

2.1.1 Indications of Reduced Mobility

Restricted arm movements relative to the body and/or the scapulae may be evident in a variety of ways:

1) The arm may be fully mobile relative to the body, with hypomobility (reduced mobility) between the scapula and the humerus, such as when the scapula is hypermobile.

2) The arm may be fully mobile relative to the body, with hypermobility (excessive mobility) between the scapula and the humerus, and reduced mobility between the scapula and the thorax, such as when the scapula is hypomobile.

3) Arm mobility relative to the body may be reduced, as when mobility is reduced at one or more joints of the shoulder girdle or at the shoulder joint itself.

4) Arm mobility relative to the body may be reduced, even though mobility is normal between the scapula and the humerus; this occurs when the latissimus dorsi, pectoralis major, or other muscles and/or structures are shortened.

2.1.2 Patient Positioning

In therapy techniques for the shoulder with the patient supine on the couch, he/she should be arranged so the couch itself does not constrain free arm movement. This may be done in two ways. First, the patient can be positioned to place the shoulder treated over the edge of the couch. Second, a small, firm cushion or other support may be placed between the patient's scapulae.

Throughout treatment, the patient should keep his/her chin tucked in to stabilize the neck and thus protect the cervical spine. So the therapist must instruct the patient to tuck his/her chin in before starting treatment, and must watch to assure that the tuck is maintained throughout the treatment.

Some therapy techniques with the patient supine require that the hips and the knees be flexed. If necessary, the foot sector of the couch may be raised to help the patient maintain these flexes.

2.1.3 Restrictions, Muscles and Therapies

The muscles which may restrict movement at the shoulder are listed in Table 2-1, along with the applicable therapies, indexed by manual section number and page. For the compound movements, some muscles listed may restrict only one or two components of the movement, but are listed as they act in the movement. Muscle actions are listed in Table 2-2.

In all cases, restriction at the shoulder may be regarded as affecting arm motion relative to the body, or conversely, body motion in the opposite direction relative to a stable arm. The various restrictions possible are listed in Movement Restriction Tables 10.1 and 10.2 (pp. 165-166).

TABLE 2.1 Restrictions at the shoulder

SECTION	MOVEMENT RESTRICTED	RESTRICTING MUSCLE(S)	THERAPY	Number	Page
2.2	*Flexion*	Pectoralis major, abdomnial part		2.2.1A, 2.2.1B	18, 19
		sternocostal part		2.2.2A, 2.2.2B	20, 21
		clavicular part		2.2.3A, 2.2.3B	22, 23
		Latissimus dorsi		2.2.4A, 2.2.4B	24, 25
		Teres major		2.2.5	26
		Pectoralis minor		2.2.6	27
		Subclavius		2.2.7	28
		Deltoid, spinal part		2.3.1	29
		Triceps brachii, long head		2.3.6A, 2.3.6B	35, 36
		Levator scapulae		2.12.2A-C	45-47
		Trapezius		2.3.4	32
		Teres minor		2.3.2	30
		Spinalis group		Volume II	
2.3	*Flexion, abduction and medial rotation*	Deltoid, spinal part		2.3.1	29
		Teres minor		2.3.2	30
		Infraspinatus		2.3.3	31
		Trapezius, transverse part		2.3.4	32
		Rombodei major and minor		2.3.5A, 2.3.5B	33, 34
		Triceps brachii, long head		2.3.6A, 2.3.6B	35, 36
2.4	*Flexion abduction and lateral rotation*	Pectoralis major		2.2.1-2.2.3	18-23
		Pectoralis minor		2.2.6	27
		Latissimus dorsi		2.2.4	24, 25
		Teres major		2.2.5	26
		Infraspinatus		2.3.3	31
		Subscapularis		2.11.3	43
2.5	*Flexion, adduction and medial rotation*	Teres minor		2.3.2	30
		Infraspinatus		2.3.3	31
2.6	*Flexion, adduction and lateral rotation*	Pectoralis major		2.2.1-2.2.3	18-23
		Pectoralis minor		2.2.6	27
		Latissimus dorsi		2.2.4	24, 25
		Teres major		2.2.5	26
		Subscapularis		2.11.3	43
		Coracobrachialis		2.11.1	41
		Biceps brachii, short head		2.11.2	42
		Deltoid, clavicular part		2.11.1	41
2.7	*Extension*	Trapezius		2.3.4, 2.8.1, 2.12.1	32, 37 44
		Serratus anterior		2.8.2	38
		Deltoid, clavicular part		2.11.1	41
		Coracobrachialis		2.11.1	41
		Pectoralis major		2.2.1-2.2.3	18-23
		Biceps brachii, short head		2.11.2	42

2.8	*Extension, adduction and medial rotation*	Pectoralis major	**2.2.1-2.2.3**	18-23
		Deltoid, clavicular part	**2.11.1**	41
		Coracobrachialis	**2.11.1**	41
		Biceps brachii, short head	**2.11.2**	42
		Teres minor	**2.3.2**	30
		Infraspinatus	**2.3.3**	31
		Trapezius, ascending part	**2.8.1**	37
		Serratus anterior	**2.8.2**	38
2.9	*Extension, adduction and lateral rotation*	Pectoralis major	**2.2.1-2.2.3**	18-23
		Deltoid, clavicular part	**2.11.1**	41
		Deltoid, acromial part	**2.9.2**	40
		Biceps brachii	**2.9.1**	39
		Supraspinatus	**2.9.2**	40
2.10	*Extension, abduction and medial rotation*	Deltoid, clavicular part	**2.11.1**	41
		Pectoralis major	**2.2.1-2.2.3**	18-23
		Coracobrachialis	**2.11.1**	41
		Biceps brachii, short head	**2.11.2**	42
		Biceps brachii, long head	**2.9.1**	39
		Serratus anterior	**2.8.2**	38
		Teres minor	**2.3.2**	30
		Infraspinatus	**2.3.3**	31
2.11	*Extension, abduction and lateral rotation*	Pectoralis major	**2.2.1-2.2.3**	18-23
		Deltoid, clavicular part	**2.11.1**	41
		Coracobrachialis	**2.11.1**	41
		Subscapularis	**2.11.3**	42
2.12	*Depression of the shoulder girdle*	Trapezius, descending part	**2.12.1**	44
		Levator scapulae	**2.12.2**	42
2.13	*Elevation of the shoulder girdle*	Pectoralis major	**2.2.1-2.2.3**	18-23
		Pectoralis minor	**2.2.6**	27
		Latissimus dorsi	**2.2.4**	24, 25
		Serratus anterior	**2.8.2**	38
		Subclavius	**2.2.7**	28
		Trapezius	**2.3.4, 2.8.1,**	32, 37
			2.12.1	44

TABLE 2.2 Actions of muscles which may restrict movements at the shoulder.

MUSCLE	ACTION
Muscles of the shoulder and the shoulder girdle	
Pectoralis major	Adducts and medially rotates at shoulder. Has a short extending action when shoulder is flexed. Has a short flexing action when shoulder is extended. Adducts arm in a transverse plane in relation to the body.
Pectoralis minor	Depresses raised shoulder. Pull shoulder ventrally and caudally. Assists in elevating upper ribs when raised shoulder is stable.
Latissimus dorsi	Extends, adducts and medially rotates at shoulder. Depresses shoulder girdle.
Teres major	Extends, adducts and medially rotates arm relative to scapula.
Subclavius	Depresses and stabilizes clavicle during movements of shoulder. Lifts first rib when raised shoulder is stable.
Deltoid, spinal part	Extends, adducts and laterally rotates at shoulder.
acromial part	Abducts at shoulder.
clavicular part	Flexes, medially rotates and adducts at shoulder.
Teres minor	Laterally rotates and extends at shoulder.
Infraspinatus	Laterally rotates at shoulder.
Trapezius, transverse part	Pulls scapula medially.
ascending part	Pulls shoulder girdle caudally. Laterally rotates inferior angle of scapula.
descending part	Raises shoulder girdle (when the head and neck are stable). Laterally flexes head and neck while simultaneously rotating head to opposite side (when the shoulder is stable). Extends neck when acting bilaterally.
Rhomboidei	Pulls scapulae cranially and medially while medially rotating inferior angle of scapula.
Serratus anterior	Moves scapula laterally and vetrally on rib cage. Rotates scapula so that glenoid cavity points laterally, ventrally, and slightly cranially in abducting and flexing at shoulder.
Supraspinatus	Abducts at the shoulder - also laterally or medially rotates (depending on the position of the shoulder).
Levator scapulae	Raises shoulder girdle (when head and neck are stable). Laterally flexes and rotates neck to same side (when scapula is stable). Extends neck when acting bilaterally.
Subscapularis	Medially rotates at shoulder.
Muscles of the upper arm	
Biceps brachii long head	Abducts and medially rotates at shoulder. Flexes at elbow. Supinates forearm.
Biceps brachii short head	Adducts and flexes at shoulder. Flexes at elbow. Supinates forearm.
Coracobrachialis	Flexes, medially rotates and adducts at shoulder.
Triceps brachii long head	Extends at elbow. Adducts and extends at shoulder.

2.2.1A. Therapy for the **pectoralis major, abdominal part.** *Bilateral stretching.*

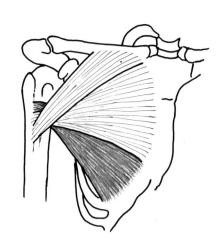

Starting Position: P: Supine on couch; knees and hips flexed to stabilize lumbar and thoracic regions and to prevent lumbar spine lordosis; head of couch lowered; small, firm cushion may be placed between scapulae to permit maximum shoulder movement; thorax stabilized to couch with a belt; chin tucked in to protect cervical spine. T: Standing at head of couch.

Grip: Using both hands, T grips medial sides of P's arms just above the elbows and holds them flexed and fully laterally rotated at the shoulders. (If P is very strong, T grips just above P's wrists).

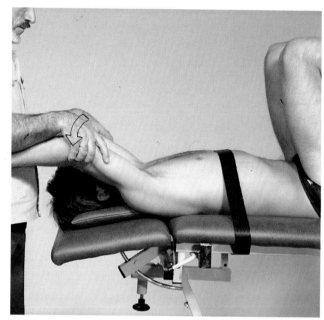

Fig. 1 a. Starting Position.

Procedure: Using this grip, T gradually and fully *flexes* at P's shoulders.

Stimulation of Antagonists: T reverses grip (to under P's arms), asks P to flex arms, and then resists the flexing to stimulate P's antagonists.

Notes: Stretching should always begin from the position where movement is most restricted.

P's shoulder joints are better protected and stretching is most effective if T applies traction to P's arms as P flexes them.

The **latissimus dorsi, teres major** and **pectoralis minor** are also stretched in this procedure.

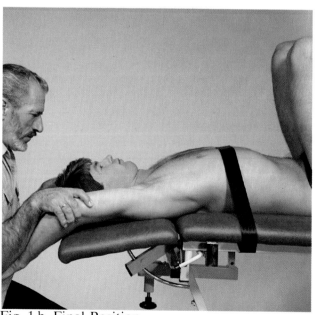

Fig. 1 b. Final Position.

2.2.1B.   Therapy for the **pectoralis major, abdominal part.** *Unilateral stretching.*

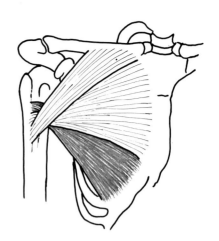

Starting Position P: Supine; knees and hips flexed to stabilize lumbar and thoracic regions and to prevent lumbar spine lordosis; small firm cushion may be placed between scapulae to permit maximum shoulder movement; support under head and neck; chin tucked in to protect cervical spine; arm flexed above head. T: Standing oblique to P's right side, facing P's head.

Grip: T's left hand grips medial side of P's upper arm just above the elbow and holds it flexed and fully laterally rotated at the shoulder. P's forearm lies along T's forearm with P's right hand on the medial side of T's upper arm. T's right hand stabilizes P's thorax.

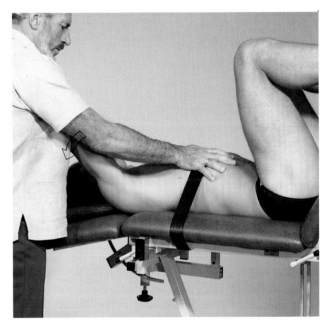

Fig. 2 a. Starting Position.

Procedure: Using this grip, T gradually and fully *flexes* at P's shoulder.

Stimulation of Antagonists: T reverses grip on P's arm, asks P to move further in the direction of stretching, and then resists that movement to stimulate P's antagonists.

Notes: Stabilization of the thorax is easier if both sides are stretched simultaneously (see page 18).

The **latissimus dorsi, teres major** and **pectoralis minor** are also stretched in this procedure.

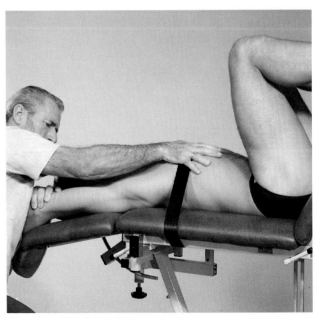

Fig. 2 b. Final Position.

19

2.2.2A.   Therapy for the **pectoralis major, sternocostal part.** *Bilateral stretching.*

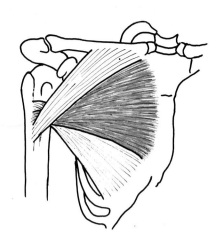

Starting Position: P: Supine; knees and hips flexed to stabilize lumbar and thoracic regions and to prevent lumbar spine lordosis; small, firm cushion may be placed between scapulae to permit maximum shoulder movement; thorax stabilized to couch with a belt; support under head and neck; chin tucked in to protect cervical spine; arms flexed above head. T: Standing at head of couch.

Grip: Using both hands, T grips P's elbows and forearms. T holds P's arms flexed and fully laterally rotated in the position of greatest restriction, between 90° abduction and full flexion. (If P is very strong, T can grip P's lower arms just above the wrists).

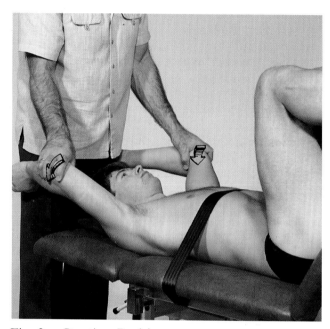

Fig. 3 a. Starting Position.

Procedure: Using this grip, T gradually and fully *flexes* at P's shoulders.

Stimulation of Antagonists: T reverses grip (to under P's arms). T then asks P to move arms further in the direction of stretching, and resists that movement to stimulate P's antagonists.

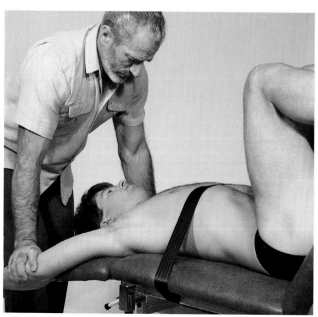

Fig. 3 b. Final Position.

2.2.2B. Therapy for the **pectoralis major, sternocostal part.** *Unilateral stretching.*

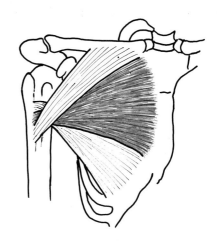

Starting Position: P: Supine; knees and hips flexed to stabilize lumbar and thoracic regions and to prevent lumbar spine lordosis; small, firm cushion may be placed between scapulae to permit maximum shoulder movement; support under head and neck; chin tucked in to protect cervical spine; thorax stabilized to couch with a belt; arm flexed above head. T: Standing with left side towards right side of P's head.

Grip: T's left hand grips medial side of P's upper arm just above the elbow. T holds P's arm flexed and fully laterally rotated in the position of greatest restriction, between full flexion and 90° abduction at the shoulder. P's forearm lies along T's forearm with P's hand against the medial side of T's upper arm. T's right hand presses against P's sternum to stabilize the thorax.

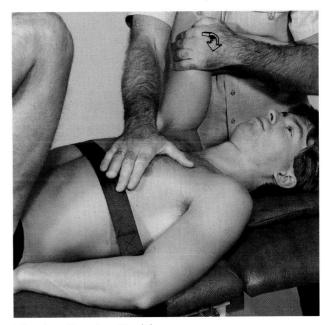

Fig. 4 a. Starting Position.

Procedure: Using this grip, T gradually and fully *flexes* at P's shoulder.

Stimulation of Antagonists: T reverses left-hand grip (to under P's arm). T then asks P to move further in the direction of stretching, and resists that movement to stimulate P's antagonists.

Note: Stabilization of the thorax is easier if both sides are stretched simultaneously, see therapy 2.2.2A., p. 20.

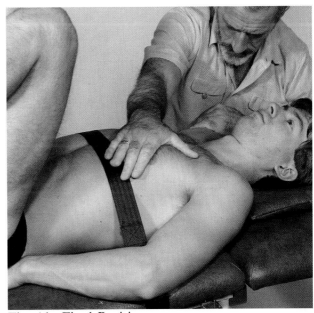

Fig. 4 b. Final Position.

2.2.3A. Therapy for the **pectoralis major, clavicular part.** *Bilateral stretching.*

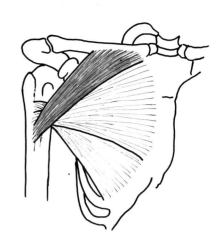

Starting Position: P: Supine; knees and hips flexed to stabilize lumbar and thoracic regions and to prevent lumbar spine lordosis; small, firm cushion may be placed between scapulae to permit maximum shoulder movement; thorax stabilized to couch with a belt; support under head and neck; chin tucked in to protect cervical spine; arms flexed above head. T: Standing at head of couch.

Grip: Using both hands, T grips medial sides of P's upper arms at the elbows. T holds P's arms flexed, fully laterally rotated and in approximately 90° abduction at the shoulders with P's elbows flexed 90°. (If P is very strong, T can grip P's forearms or hands. If T's hands are large enough, he/she may be able to grip P's elbows and forearms to maintain maximal lateral rotation).

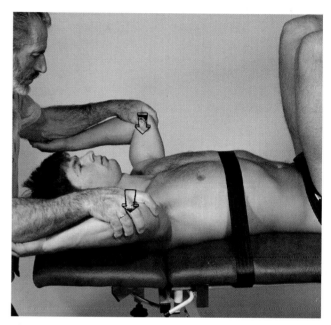

Fig. 5 a. Starting Position.

Procedure: Using this grip, T gradually and fully *abducts* at P's shoulders.

Stimulation of Antagonists: T reverses grip (to under P's arms). T then asks P to move further in the direction of stretching, and resists that movement to stimulate P's antagonists.

Note: The **pectoralis major** may also be bilaterally stretched with P sitting. P's back should be supported (with a chair, a cushion, T's knee, etc.) with hips fully flexed to stabilize the pelvis and protect the lumbar spine. T stretches by using the above technique.

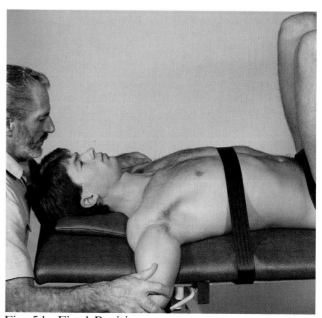

Fig. 5 b. Final Position.

22

2.2.3B. Therapy for the **pectoralis major, clavicular part.** *Unilateral stretching.*

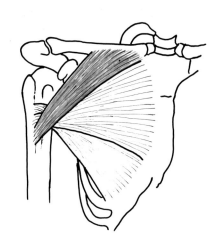

Starting Position: P: Supine; knees and hips flexed to stabilize lumbar and thoracic regions and to prevent lumbar spine lordosis; small, firm cushion may be placed between scapulae to permit maximum shoulder movement; thorax stabilized to couch with a belt; support under head and neck; chin tucked in to protect cervical spine; arm flexed above head. T: Standing facing P's right shoulder.

Grip: T's right hand grips medial side of P's upper arm just above the elbow. T holds P's arm flexed, fully laterally rotated and in less than 90° abduction in the position where maximally stretched. P's forearm lies along T's forearm with P's hand against the medial side of T's upper arm. T's left hand is placed over P's manubrium sternum and left clavicle to stabilize the thorax.

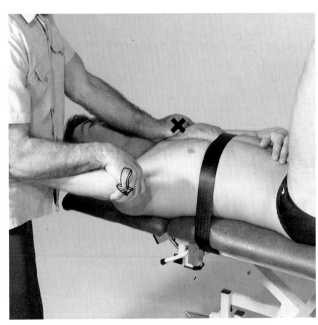

Fig. 6 a. Starting Position.

Procedure: Using this grip, T gradually and fully *abducts* at P's shoulder.

Stimulation of Antagonists: T reverses right-hand grip (to under P's arm). T then asks P to move further in the direction of stretching, and resists that movement to stimulate P's antagonists.

Note: Stabilization of the thorax is easier if both sides are stretched simultaneously, see therapy 2.2.3A, p. 22.

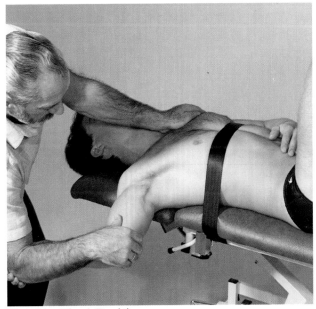

Fig. 6 b. Final Position.

2.2.4A. Therapy for the **latissimus dorsi**.
Bilateral stretching.

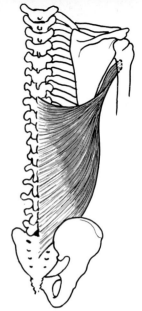

Starting Position: P: Supine; knees and hips flexed to stabilize lumbar and thoracic regions and to prevent lumbar spine lordosis; head of couch lowered and small, firm cushion may be placed between scapulae to permit maximum shoulder movement; abdomen stabilized to couch with a belt; chin tucked in to protect cervical spine; arms flexed above head. T: Standing at head of couch.

Grip: Using both hands, T grips P's upper arms from the medial aspect at the elbows. T holds P's arms flexed and in full lateral rotation at the shoulders. (If P is very strong, T can grip P's forearms or hands for better leverage).

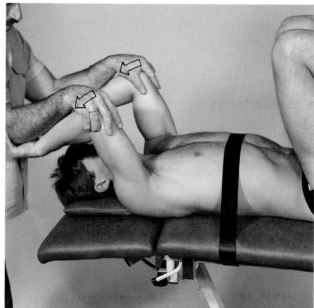

Fig. 7 a. Starting Position.

Procedure: Using this grip, T gradually and fully *flexes* at P's shoulders.

Stimulation of Antagonists: T reverses grip (to under P's arms). T then asks P to move further in the direction of stretching, and resists that movement to stimulate P's antagonists.

Notes: P's shoulder joints are better protected and stretching is most effective if T applies traction to P's arms as they are flexed.

The lumbar spine can be better stabilized by fully flexing P's hips and knees and moving the belt to the dorsal aspect of P's thighs.

The **pectoralis major and minor** and the **teres major** are also stretched in this procedure.

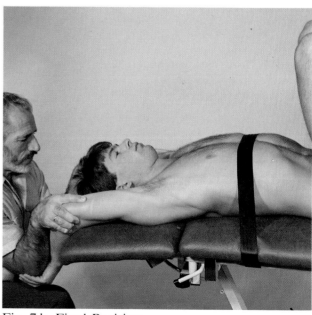

Fig. 7 b. Final Position.

2.2.4B. Therapy for the **latissimus dorsi.** *Unilateral stretching.*

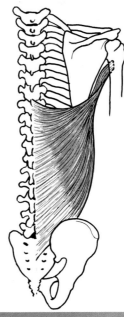

Starting Position: P: Supine; knees and hips flexed to stabilize lumbar and thoracic regions and to prevent lumbar spine lordosis; small, firm cushion may be placed between scapulae to permit maximum shoulder movement; hips and thorax stabilized with a belt; support under head and neck; chin tucked in to protect cervical spine; arm flexed above head. T: Standing at head of couch, facing oblique to P's right side.

Grip:. T's left hand grips medial side of P's upper arm just above the elbow. T holds P's arm flexed and fully laterally rotated at the shoulder. P's forearm lies along T's forearm with P's hand against the medial side of T's upper arm. T's right hand stabilizes the lower right side of P's thorax. (If P is very strong, T's left hand can grip P's right hand while T's right hand grips just above P's elbow).

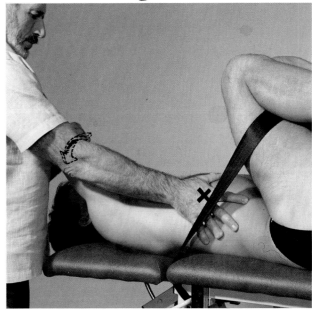

Fig. 8 a. Starting Position.

Procedure: Using this grip, T gradually and fully *flexes* and *laterally rotates* at P's shoulder and simultaneously applies traction to P's arm while moving it dorsally.

Stimulation of Antagonists: T reverses left-hand grip (to under P's arm). T then asks P to move further in the direction of stretching, and resists that movement to stimulate P's antagonists.

Note: Stabilization of the thorax is easier if both sides are stretched simultaneously, see therapy 2.2.4A, p. 24.

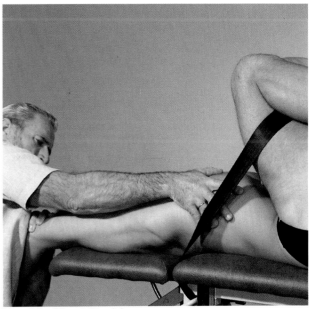

Fig. 8 b. Final Position.

2.2.5.   Therapy for the **teres major.**

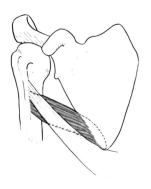

Starting Position: P: Supine; knees and hips flexed to stabilize lumbar and thoracic regions and to prevent lumbar spine lordosis; small, firm cushion may be placed between scapulae to permit maximum shoulder movement; support under head and neck; chin tucked in to protect cervical spine; arm flexed above head. T: Standing at head of couch, facing oblique to P's right side.

Grip: T's left hand grips the medial side of P's upper arm just above the elbow. T holds P's arm flexed and laterally rotated at the shoulder. P's forearm lies along T's forearm with P's right hand against the medial side of T's upper arm. T stabilizes P's scapula, using right hand to stabilize the lateral border.

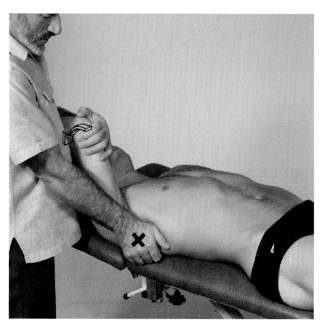

Fig. 9 a. Starting Position.

Procedure: Using this grip, T gradually and fully *flexes* and *laterally* rotates at P's shoulder.

Stimulation of Antagonists: T reverses left-hand grip to under P's arm. T then asks P to move further in the direction of stretching, and resists that movement to stimulate P's antagonists.

Note: *Not* applying traction to P's arm when flexing partly prevents involving the **latissimus dorsi** and the **pectoralis major.**

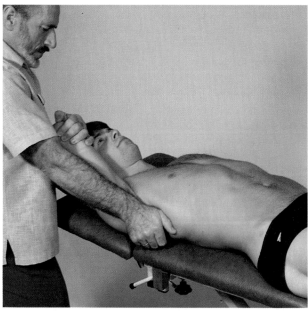

Fig. 9 b. Final Position.

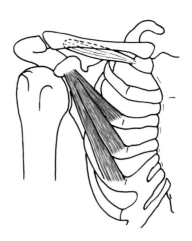

Starting Position: P: Supine; scapula over side of couch; arm in lateral rotation, adduction and less than 90° flexion at the shoulder; elbow flexed. T: Standing at P's right side, facing P's head.

Grip: T's left hand grips P's right shoulder. T's right hand grips proximal to P's wrist with P's forearm supported against T's chest.

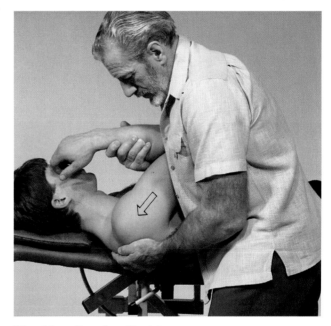

Fig. 10 a. Starting Position.

Procedure: Using this grip, T gradually and maximally moves P's shoulder girdle by pressing *cranially* and *dorsally* against P's forearm and elbow down through the line of the upper arm.

Stimulation of Antagonists: T retains grip. T then asks P to move further in the direction of stretching, and resists that movement to stimulate P's antagonists.

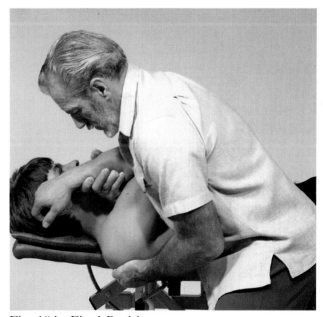

Fig. 10 b. Final Position.

2.2.7.   Therapy for the **subclavius.**

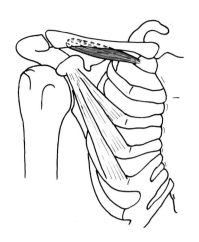

Starting Position: P: Sitting; elbow flexed with forearm against thorax; back stabilized against T's chest. T: Standing behind P.

Grip: With arms around P, T uses both hands to grip P's right elbow and forearm.

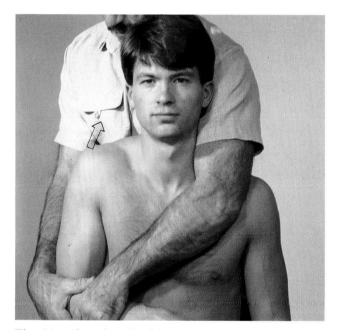

Fig. 11 a. Starting Position.

Procedure: Using this grip, T gradually and maximally moves P's shoulder girdle *cranially* by pulling up against the elbow.

Stimulation of Antagonists: T moves both hands to P's shoulder. T then asks P to move further in the direction of stretching, and resists that movement to stimulate P's antagonists.

Notes: During treatment, P should exhale when the shoulder pulled cranially; this moves the first rib caudally. (See Volume II, The Spine and Temporomandibular Joint).

If strong enough, T can use right hand to grip P's elbow, and left hand to support P's left shoulder.

The **deltoid, acromial part** and the **supraspinatus** are also stretched in this procedure. (To avoid the stretching of these muscles, P's right arm should be abducted during the stretching.)

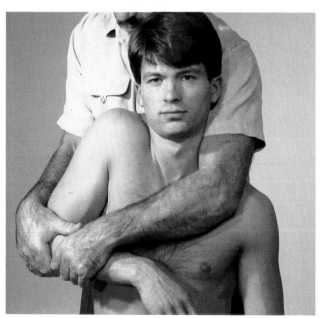

Fig. 11 b. Final Position.

28

2.3.1.   Therapy for the **deltoid, spinal part.**

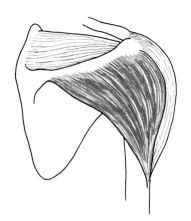

Starting Position: P: Supine; knees and hips flexed; arm flexed approximately 90° at shoulder. T: Standing at head of couch, facing oblique to P's left side.

Grip: T's right hand grips the dorsal side of P's elbow. The dorsal side of P's forearm should lie along the medial side of T's forearm. T's left hand stabilizes the lateral border of P's right scapula.

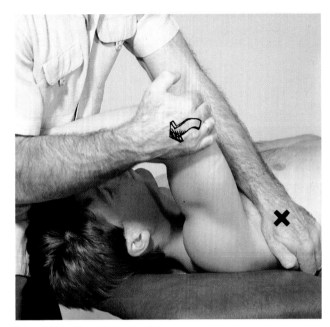

Fig. 12 a. Starting Position.

Procedure: Using this grip, T gradually and fully *flexes*, *adducts* (over and behind P's head) and *medially rotates* at P's shoulder.

Stimulation of Antagonists: T reverses right-hand grip to ventral side of elbow. T then asks P to move further in the direction of stretching, and resists that movement to stimulate P's antagonists.

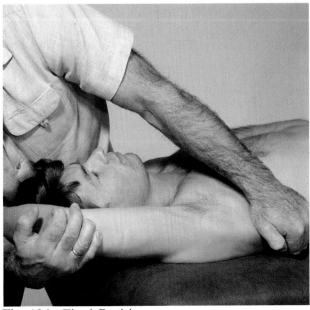

Fig. 12 b. Final Position.

2.3.2.   Therapy for the **teres minor**.

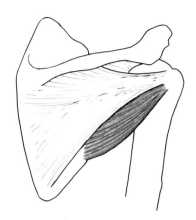

Starting Position: P: Sitting; right, upper arm fully flexed and adducted at shoulder; elbow flexed approximately 90°. T: Standing behind P.

Grip: T's left hand grips P's forearm just above the wrist. T's right hand grips P's upper arm just above the elbow.

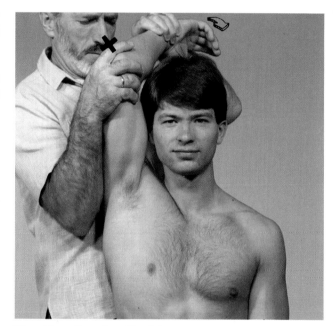

Fig. 13 a. Starting Position.

Procedure: Using this grip, T gradually rotates P's arm until full *medial rotation* is attained at the shoulder.

Stimulation of Antagonists: T reverses left-hand grip to other side of forearm. T then asks P to move further in the direction of stretching, and resists that movement to stimulate P's antagonists.

Note: The **deltoid, spinal part** and the **infraspinatus** are also stretched in this procedure.

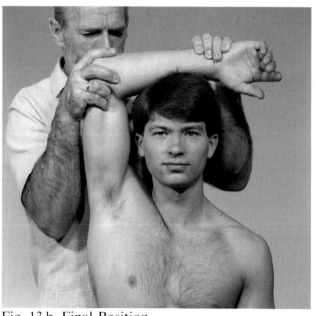

Fig. 13 b. Final Position.

2.3.3. Therapy for the **infraspinatus.**

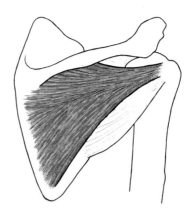

Starting Position: P: Supine; arm abducted approximately 90° and elbow flexed 90°. T: Standing at head of couch.

Grip: T's right hand grips P's forearm just above the wrist. T's left hand steadies P's shoulder at the ventral side.

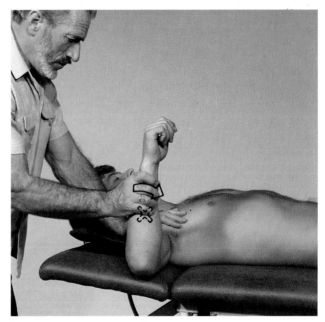

Fig. 14 a. Starting Position.

Procedure: Using this grip, T gradually rotates P's arm until full *medial rotation* is attained at the shoulder.

Stimulation of Antagonists: T retains grip. T then asks P to move further in the direction of stretching, and resists that movement to stimulate P's antagonists.

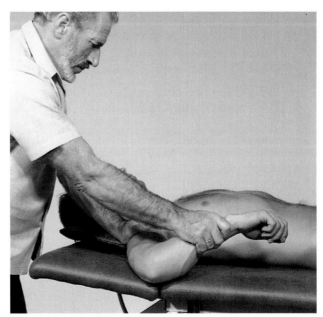

Fig. 14 b. Final Position.

2.3.4. Therapy for the **trapezius, transverse part.**

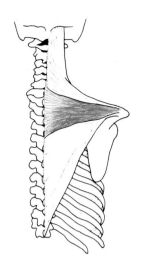

Starting Position: P: Lying on left side; right shoulder flexed approximately 90°. T: Standing, left side against P's chest and abdomen.

Grip: T's left hand grips P's scapula dorsally and along the medial border. T's right hand grips P's upper arm.

Procedure: Using this grip, T gradually and maximally pushes in a *lateral* and *ventral* direction against P's scapula.

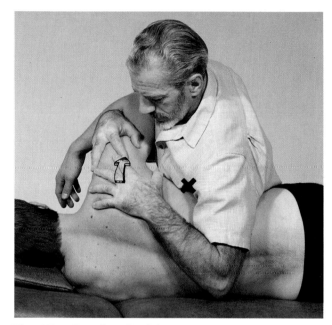

Fig. 15 a. Starting Position.

Stimulation of Antagonists: T retains right-hand grip. T then asks P to move further in the direction of stretching, and resists that movement to stimulate P's antagonists.

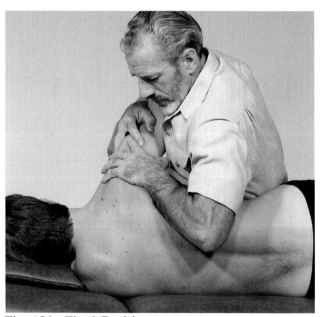

Fig. 15 b. Final Position.

2.3.5A. Therapy for the **rhomboidei major and minor.** *P prone.*

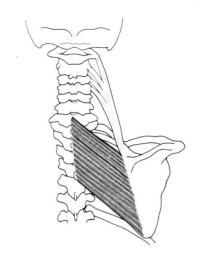

Starting Position: P: Prone; right arm hanging free over edge of couch. T: Standing at head of couch, to P's left.

Grip: T's left hand on P's right scapula, its thenar eminence along the scapula medial border. T's right hand steadies P's thorax from P's left.

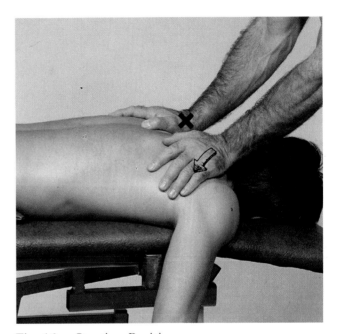

Fig. 16 a. Starting Position.

Procedure: Using this grip, T gradually and maximally pushes in a *lateral*, *ventral* and *caudal* direction against P's scapula.

Stimulation of Antagonists: T moves left-hand grip to ventral side of P's right shoulder, and uses right hand to stabilize P's thorax on right side. T then asks P to move further in the direction of stretching, and resists that movement to stimulate P's antagonists.

Note: The **trapezius, transverse part** is also stretched in this procedure.

If the prone position is inconvenient or uncomfortable, P may be treated lying on side; see following technique, therapy 2.3.5B, p. 34.

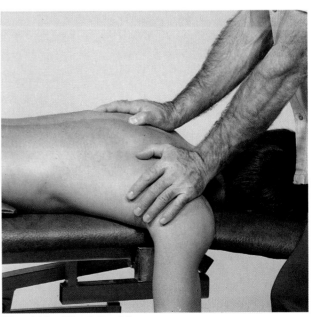

Fig. 16 b. Final Position.

33

2.3.5B. Therapy for the **rhomboidei major and minor.** *P lying on side.*

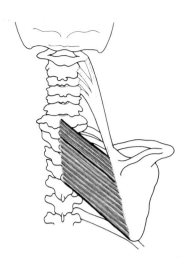

Starting Position: P: Lying on left side; right shoulder flexed approximately 90°. T: Standing and half sitting on couch, with left side against P's abdomen and chest.

Grip: T's left hand grips P's scapula dorsally along the medial border. T's right hand grips P's upper arm at the shoulder.

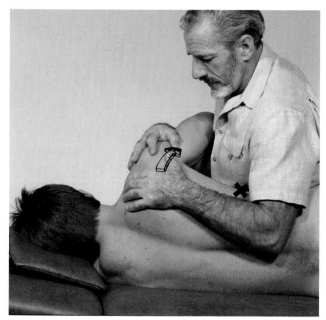

Fig. 17 a. Starting Position.

Procedure: Using this grip, T gradually and maximally pushes in a *lateral*, *ventral* and *caudal* direction against P's scapula.

Stimulation of Antagonists: T retains grip. T then asks P to move further in the direction of stretching, and resists that movement to stimulate P's antagonists.

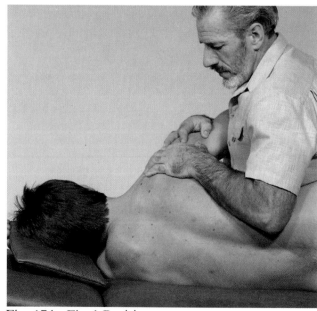

Fig. 17 b. Final Position.

2.3.6A. Therapy for the **triceps brachii, long head.**

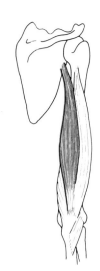

Starting Position: P: Sitting; shoulder fully flexed and adducted with elbow flexed. T: Standing facing P's left side, or behind P if P's shoulder has restricted flexion.

Grip: T's right hand grips P's forearm above the wrist. T's left hand stabilizes lateral side of P's shoulder. (When T stands behind P, T's left hand grips P's forearm above the wrist. T's right hand stabilizes P's upper arm above the elbow).

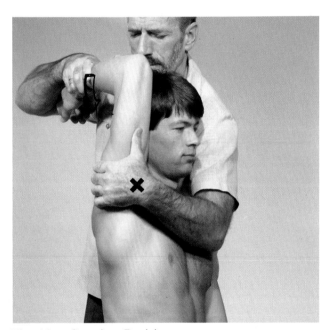

Fig. 18 a. Starting Position.

Procedure: Using this grip, T gradually and fully *flexes* at P's elbow.

Stimulation of Antagonists: T retains grip. T then asks P to move further in the direction of stretching, and resists that movement to stimulate P's antagonists.

Note: If T has difficulty stabilizing P, procedure may be performed with P lying on side; see following technique, therapy 2.3.6B, p. 36.

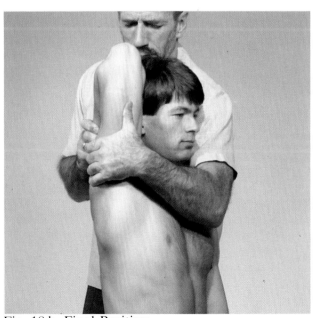

Fig. 18 b. Final Position.

2.3.6B. Therapy for the **triceps brachii, long head.** *P lying on side.*

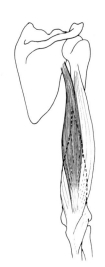

Starting Position: P: Lying on right side; shoulder fully flexed; head of couch raised so shoulder is also fully adducted. T: Standing facing P from front.

Grip: T's left hand grips P's right forearm just above the wrist. T's right hand stabilizes P's shoulder from behind.

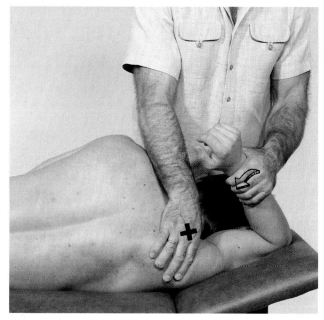

Fig. 19 a. Starting Position.

Procedure: Using this grip, T gradually and fully *flexes* at P's elbow.

Stimulation of Antagonists: T retains grip. T then asks P to move further in the direction of stretching, and resists that movement to stimulate P's antagonists.

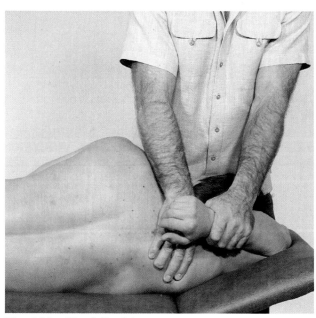

Fig. 19 b. Final Position.

36

2.8.1. Therapy for the **trapezius, ascending part.**

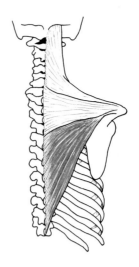

Starting Position: P: Lying on left side; right arm behind back. T: Standing, obliquely facing P.

Grip: T's left hand grips lateral border and the inferior angle of P's scapula. T's right hand grips the acromion, coracoid process and head of humerus. T's chest supports elbow.

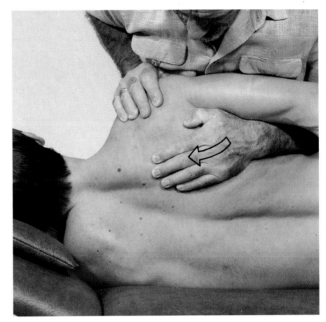
Fig. 20 a. Starting Position.

Procedure: Using this grip, T gradually and maximally moves P's scapula in a *cranial* and *medial* direction. This produces a lateral and slightly caudal rotation of the glenoid cavity.

Stimulation of Antagonists: T moves left hand to upper medial angle of scapula. T then asks P to move further in the direction of stretching, and resists that movement with left hand to stimulate P's antagonists.

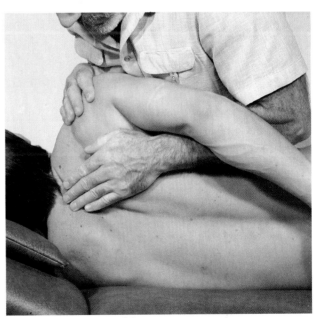
Fig. 20 b. Final Position.

2.8.2.   Therapy for the **serratus anterior**.

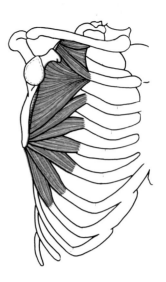

Starting Position: P: Sitting. T: Standing at P's left side, chest and abdomen stabilizing P's upper arm and shoulder.

Grip: T's right hand grips the lateral/dorsal side of P's upper arm just above the elbow, and holds the arm medially rotated and fully adducted. T's left hand grips the ventral/lateral side of P's shoulder.

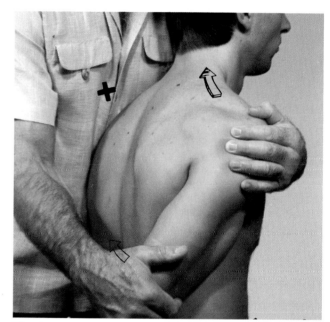

Fig. 21 a. Starting Position.

Procedure: Using this grip, T gradually and maximally moves P's scapula in a *cranial, dorsal* and *medial* direction.

Stimulation of Antagonists: T moves right hand, cupping palm over dorsal-medial side of P's elbow. T then asks P to move further in the direction of stretching, and resists that movement with right hand to stimulate P's antagonists.

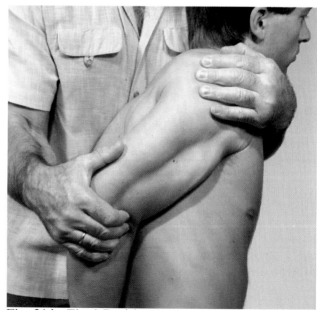

Fig. 21 b. Final Position.

2.9.1. Therapy for the **biceps brachii, long head.**

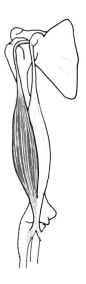

Starting Position: P: Lying on left side; right upper arm fully extended, adducted and laterally rotated at shoulder, so the sulcus intertubercularis turns laterally; elbow flexed and forearm fully pronated. T: Standing behind P, buttocks stabilizing P's lumbar and thoracic regions.

Grip: T's left hand grips P's forearm just above the wrist. T's right hand stabilizes P's upper arm just above the elbow.

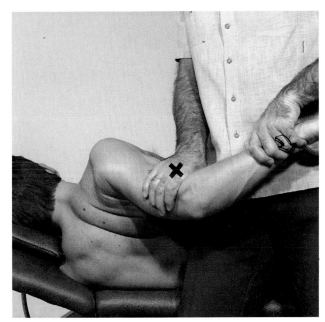

Fig. 22 a. Starting Position.

Procedure: Using this grip, T gradually and fully *extends* at P's elbow.

Stimulation of Antagonists: T retains grip. T then asks P to move further in the direction of stretching, and resists that movement with left hand to stimulate P's antagonists.

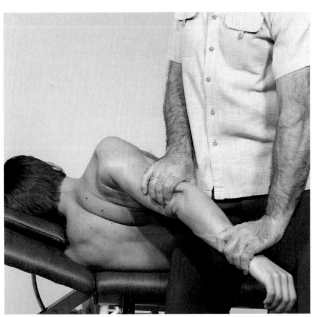

Fig. 22 b. Final Position.

2.9.2. Therapy for the **supraspinatus.**

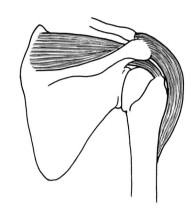

Starting Position: P: Lying on left side; right upper arm slightly abducted and extended, but not medially or laterally rotated. T: Standing behind P.

Grip: T's right hand grips P's upper arm just above the elbow. T's left forearm (or, if preferred, a firm, round cushion) is placed in P's axilla.

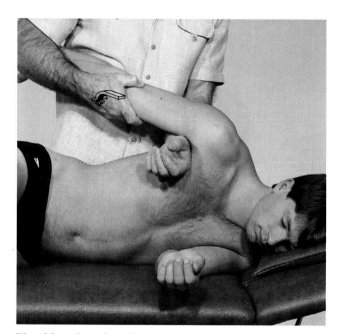

Fig. 23 a. Starting Position.

Procedure: Using this grip, T pulls against P's upper arm while pivoting at the axilla and gradually and fully *adducting* the arm behind the back.

Stimulation of Antagonists: T retains grip. T then asks P to move further in the direction of stretching, and resists that movement to stimulate P's antagonists.

Note: The **deltoid, acromial part** is also stretched in this procedure.

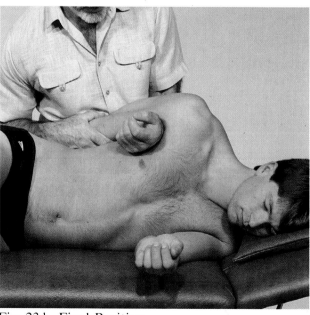

Fig. 23 b. Final Position.

2.11.1. Therapy for the **deltoid, clavicular part** and the **coracobrachialis.** *Bilateral stretching.*

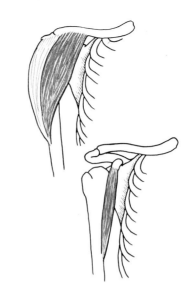

Starting Position: P: Supine; knees and hips flexed to stabilize lumbar and thoracic regions and to prevent lumbar spine lordosis; small, firm cushion may be placed between scapulae to permit maximum shoulder movement; support under head and neck; chin tucked in to protect cervical spine. T: Standing at head of couch.

Grip: Using both hands, T grips the medial sides of P's elbows, forearms against P's forearms. P's arms are abducted approximately 90° and rotated laterally. (*Note:* full abduction combined with *full* lateral rotation produces the undesirable "close packed position" at P's shoulder.)

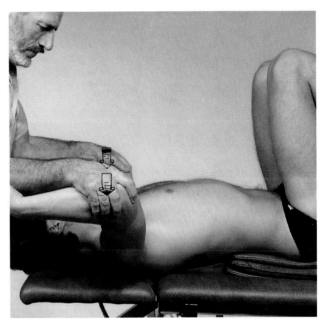

Fig. 24 a. Starting Position.

Procedure: Using this grip, T gradually and maximally moves P's arms in a *dorsal* direction.

Stimulation of Antagonists: T reverses grip to under P's arms. T then asks P to move further in the direction of stretching, and resists that movement to stimulate P's antagonists.

Notes: This procedure may also be performed with P sitting.

The **pectoralis major** and **subscapularis** are also stretched in this procedure.

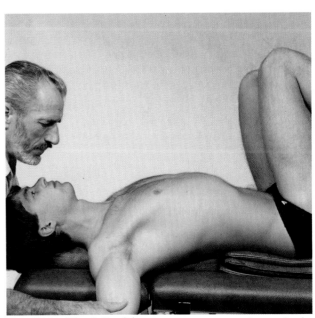

Fig. 24 b. Final Position.

2.11.2.   Therapy for the **biceps brachii, short head**.

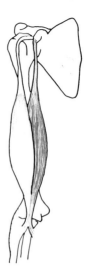

Starting Position: P: Supine; thorax stabilized to couch with a belt; upper arm fully laterally rotated and fully extended, but less than 90° abducted; elbow flexed with forearm fully pronated. T: Sitting or standing at head of couch with left side against P's right shoulder.

Grip: T's right hand grips around dorsal side of P's forearm just above the wrist. T's left hand grips dorsal-medial side of P's upper arm just above the elbow.

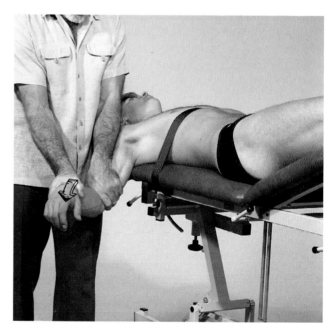

Fig. 25 a. Starting Position.

Procedure: Using this grip, T gradually and fully *extends* at P's elbow.

Stimulation of Antagonists: T retains grip. T then asks P to move further in the direction of stretching, and resists that movement to stimulate P's antagonists.

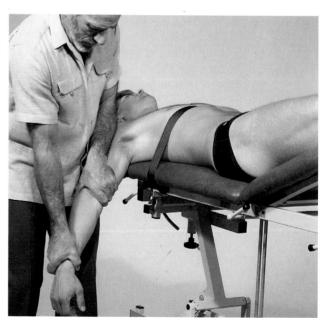

Fig. 25 b. Final Position.

42

2.11.3.   Therapy for the **subscapularis.**

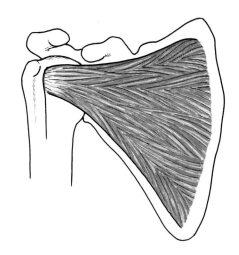

Starting Position: P: Supine; upper arm on couch with elbow flexed 90°; thorax may be stabilized to couch with a belt. T: Standing obliquely facing P's right side.

Grip: T's left hand stabilizes P's upper arm against the couch. T's right hand grips medial side of P's forearm just above the wrist.

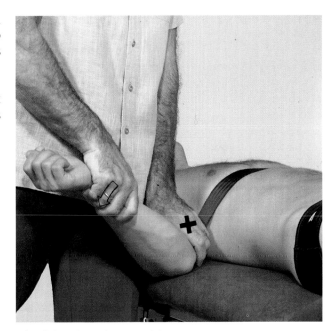

Fig. 26 a. Starting Position.

Procedure: Using this grip, T gradually rotates P's shoulder until full *lateral* rotation is attained.

Stimulation of Antagonists: T retains grip. T then asks P to move further in the direction of stretching, and resists that movement to stimulate P's antagonists.

Notes: Stretching may also be performed with P's upper arm held in various degrees of abduction.

A firm cushion placed under P's right scapula will push his shoulder girdle ventrally, thus preventing undue strain on the **pectoralis major.**

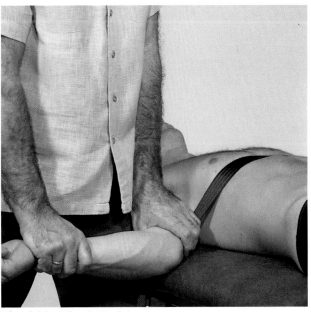

Fig. 26 b. Final Position.

2.12.1. Therapy for the **trapezius, descending part.**

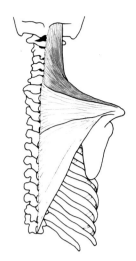

Starting Position: P: Supine; head and neck in full ventral and left lateral flexion and right rotation; shoulders at edge of head of couch. T: Standing at head of couch; left side of abdomen supports right side of P's head.

Grip: T's left hand grips the dorsal side of P's neck. P's head and neck are stabilized between T's left forearm and chest. T's right hand on P's right shoulder.

Procedure: Using this grip, T applies traction to P's neck while gradually and maximally pushing P's shoulder in a *caudal* and *dorsal* direction.

Stimulation of Antagonists: T moves right hand, cupping P's right elbow in palm. T then asks P to move further in the direction of stretching., and resists that movement to stimulate P's antagonists.

Note: Avoid any movements of P's head and neck other than the prescribed traction applied.

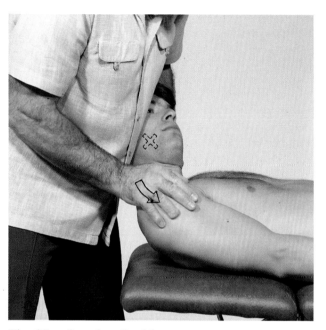

Fig. 27 a. Starting Position.

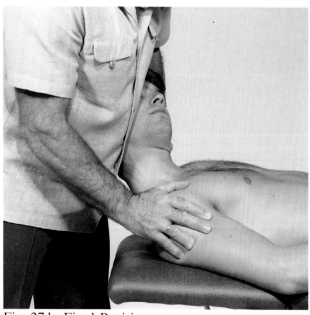

Fig. 27 b. Final Position.
(Viewed from side)

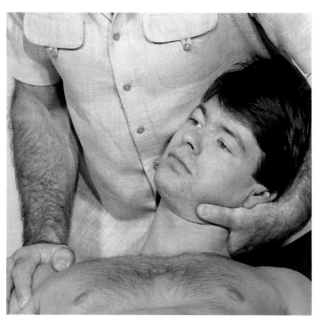

Fig. 28 Final Position.
(Viewed from below)

2.12.2A. Therapy for the **levator scapulae**.

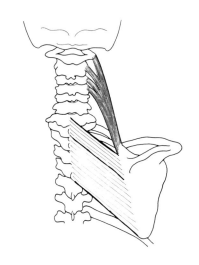

Starting Position: P: Supine; head and neck in full ventral and left lateral flexion and left rotation; shoulders at edge of head of couch; right arm fully flexed above head and abducted towards head; elbow flexed approximately 90°. T: Standing at head of couch with chest supporting right side of P's head.

Grip: T's left hand grips dorsal side of P's neck. P's head and neck are stabilized between T's left arm and thorax. P's right elbow against T's abdomen. T's right hand grips dorsal-lateral side of P's upper arm and shoulder.

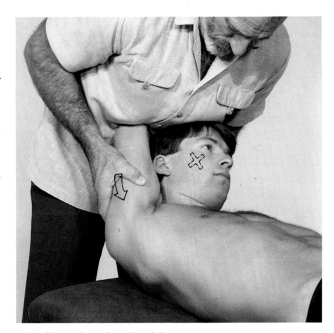

Fig. 29 a. Starting Position.

Procedure: Using this grip, T applies traction to P's neck while leaning abdomen against P's elbow. T's right hand then moves P's shoulder gradually and maximally in a *caudal* and *dorsal* direction.

Stimulation of Antagonists: T retains grip. T then asks P to move further in the direction of stretching, and resists that movement with right hand to stimulate P's antagonists.

Note: Avoid any movements of P's head and neck other than the prescribed traction applied.

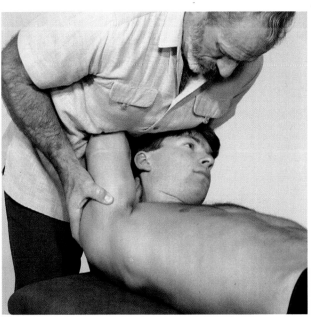

Fig. 29 b. Final Position.

2.12.2B. Therapy for the **levator scapulae.**
Alternative grip for patients with good shoulder flexion.

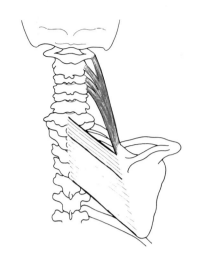

Starting Position: P: Supine; head and neck in full ventral and left lateral flexion and left rotation; shoulders at edge of head of couch; right arm fully flexed above head and abducted towards head; elbow flexed approximately 90°.

T: Standing at head of couch with chest supporting right side of P's head.
Grip: T's left hand grips dorsal side of P's neck. P's head and neck are stabilized between T's left arm and thorax. T's right hand stabilizes P's chin.

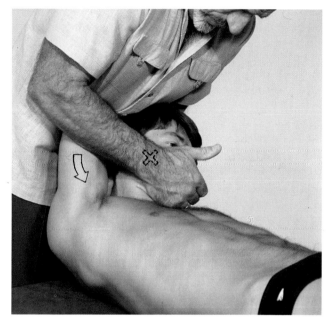

Fig. 30 a. Starting Position.

Procedure: Using this grip, T applies traction to P's neck with both hands, while leaning abdomen against P's elbow and moving P's shoulder gradually and maximally in a *caudal* and *dorsal* direction.

Stimulation of Antagonists: T moves right hand to P's upper right arm. T then asks P to move right shoulder further in the direction of stretching, and resists that movement with right hand to stimulate P's antagonists.

Note: Avoid any movements of P's head and neck other than the prescribed traction applied.

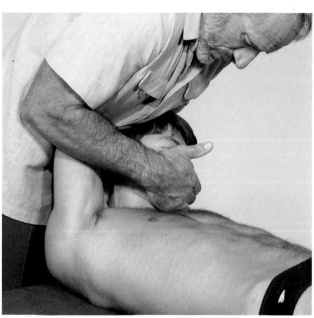

Fig. 30 b. Final Position.

2.12.2C. Therapy for the **levator scapulae.**
When P's shoulder is painful.

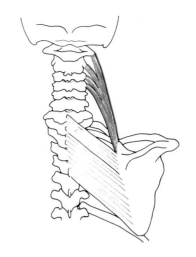

Starting Position: P: Supine; head and neck in full ventral and left lateral flexion and left rotation; on couch and not beyond edge; right arm abducted and fully laterally rotated at shoulder with upper arm resting on couch. T: Standing at head of couch, chest supporting right side of P's head.

Grip: T's left hand grips dorsal side of P's neck. P's head and neck are stabilized between T's left arm and chest. T's right hand is on the dorsal side of P's scapula with the thenar eminence against P's supraspinous fossa.

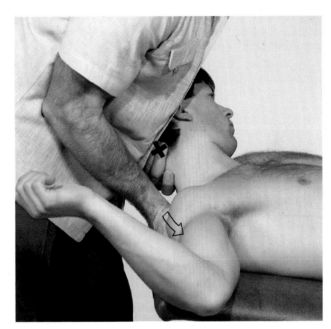

Fig. 31 a. Starting Position.

Procedure: Using this grip, T applies traction to P's neck while gradually and maximally pushing P's scapula in a *caudal* and *dorsal* direction.

Stimulation of Antagonists: T moves right hand to P's axilla. T then asks P to move right shoulder further in the direction of stretching, and resists that movement with right hand to stimulate P's antagonists.

Notes: This procedure should be used if flexing is constrained at P's shoulder and/or if stretching causes pain at the shoulder.

Avoid any movements of P's head and neck other than the traction applied.

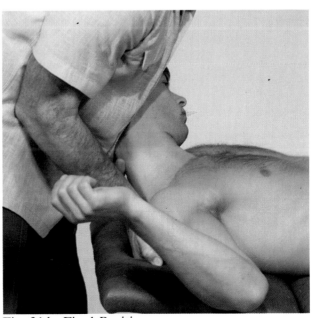

Fig. 31 b. Final Position.

3 THE ELBOW

3.1 THERAPY GUIDE

The muscles which may restrict movement at the elbow are listed in Table 3-1, along with the applicable therapies, indexed by manual section number and page. Muscle actions are listed in Table 3-2.

The various restrictions possible are listed in Movement Restriction Table 10.3 (p.167).

TABLE 3.1 Restrictions at the elbow

SECTION	MOVEMENT RESTRICTED	RESTRICTING MUSCLE(S)	THERAPY	Number	Page
3.2	*Flexion*	Triceps brachii			
		long head		2.3.6	35, 36
		medial & lateral heads		3.2.1	51
		Anconeus		3.2.1	51
3.3	*Extension and supination/pronation of forearm*	Biceps brachii		2.9.1, 2.11.2	39, 42
		Brachialis		3.3.1	52
		Brachioradialis		3.3.2	53
		Extensor carpi radialis longus		3.3.3	54
		Extensor carpi radialis brevis		3.3.4	55
		Extensor digitorum communis		3.3.5	56
		fingers simultaneously			
		middle finger individually		3.3.7	58
		Extensor indicis		3.3.6	57
		Extensor digiti minimi		3.3.8	59
		Supinator		3.3.9	60
		Extensor carpi ulnaris		3.3.10	61
		Flexor carpi ulnaris		3.3.11	62
		Flexor carpi radialis		3.3.12	63
		Flexor digitorum superficialis		3.3.13	64
		Pronator teres, humeral head		3.3.14	65
		ulnar head		3.3.15	66
		Pronator quadratus		3.3.15	66
		Palmaris longus		3.3.16	67

TABLE 3.2 Actions of muscles which may restrict movement at the elbow

MUSCLE	ACTION
Muscles of the upper arm	
Triceps brachii	
– long head	Extends at elbow. Adducts and extends at shoulder.
– medial/lateral heads	Extend at elbow.
Biceps brachii	Flexes at elbow. Supinates forearm. Long head abducts and medially rotates at shoulder; short head adducts and flexes at shoulder.
Brachialis	Flexes at elbow.
Muscles of the forearm	
Anconeus	Extends at elbow. Tightens joint capsule.
Brachioradialis	Flexes at elbow. Supinates forearm from pronated position. Pronates forearm from supinated position.
Extensor carpi radialis longus	Flexes at elbow. Supinates forearm. Dorsal and radial flexes at wrist.
Extensor carpi radialis brevis	Flexes at elbow. Supinates forearm. Dorsal flexes at wrist.
Extensor digitorum communis	Extends fingers. Flexes at elbow. Supinates forearm. Dorsal flexes at wrist.
Extensor indicis	Extends and ulnar deviates index finger. Supinates forearm. Dorsal flexes at wrist.
Extensor digiti minimi	Extends little finger. Flexes at elbow. Dorsal and ulnar flexes at wrist.
Supinator	Supinates forearm. Flexes at the elbow.
Extensor carpi ulnaris	Dorsal and ulnar flexes at wrist. Flexes at elbow. Supinates forearm.
Flexor carpi ulnaris	Flexes at elbow. Pronates forearm. Volar and ulnar flexes at wrist.
Flexor carpi radialis	Flexes at elbow. Pronates forearm. Volar and radial flexes at wrist.
Flexor digitorum superficialis	Flexes the fingers (including at the proximal interphalangeal joints). Flexes at the elbow. Volar flexes at wrist.
Pronator teres, humeral head	Pronates forearm. Flexes at elbow.
ulnar head	Pronates forearm.
Pronator quadratus	Pronates forearm.
Palmaris longus	Flexes at elbow. Pronates forearm. Volar flexes at wrist.

NOTE: Actions describes in terms most relevant to manual therapy. Cross-reference to terms often used in anatomy texts:

Ulnar flexion: towards ulna, corresponds to adduction (usually of hand)
Radial flexion: towards radius, corresponds to abduction (usually of hand)
Volar flexion: towards palm, corresponds to flexion of hand
Dorsal flexion: towards back of hand, corresponds to extension of hand

3.2.1. Therapy for the **triceps brachii, medial and lateral heads** and the **anconeus.**

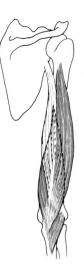

Starting Position: P: Supine; arm slightly abducted with elbow flexed. T: Standing, right side against P.

Grip: T's left hand grips dorsal side of P's forearm just above wrist. T's right hand stabilizes P's upper arm just below the shoulder.

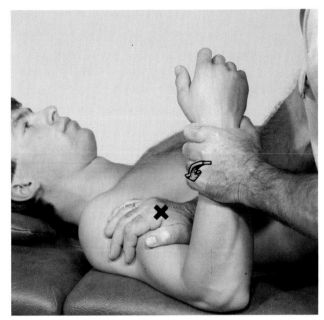
Fig. 32 a. Starting Position.

Procedure: Using this grip, T gradually and fully *flexes* at P's elbow.

Stimulation of Antagonists: T retains grip. T then asks P to move further in the direction of stretching, and resists that movement to stimulate P's antagonists.

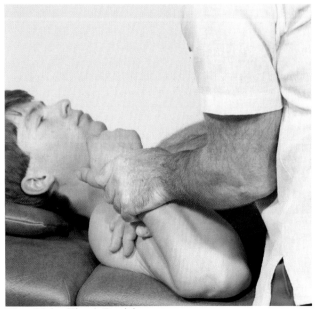
Fig. 32 b. Final Position.

3.3.1. Therapy for the **brachialis**.

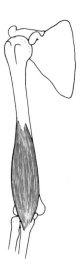

Starting Position: P: Supine; right arm and forearm both flexed approximately 90° to relax biceps. T: Standing facing P's right side.

Grip: T's right hand grips medial side of P's forearm just above wrist. T's left hand stabilizes P's upper arm at dorsal side just above the elbow.

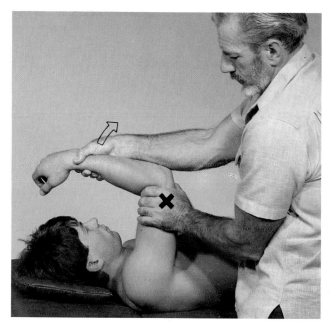

Fig. 33 a. Starting Position.

Procedure: Using this grip, T gradually and fully *extends* at P's elbow.

Stimulation of Antagonists: T retains grip. T then asks P to continue extending forearm, and resists that extension with right arm (T's left hand still stabilizes P's arm) to stimulate P's antagonists.

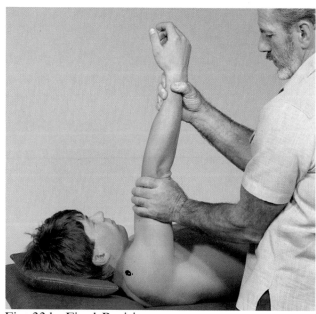

Fig. 33 b. Final Position.

3.3.2.   Therapy for the **brachioradialis.**

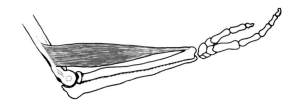

Starting Position: P: Supine; right arm flexed approximately 90° and fully medially rotated; forearm flexed and fully pronated. T: standing facing P's right side.

Grip: T's right hand grips medial side of P's forearm just above the wrist. T's left hand stabilizes P's upper arm at the lateral side just above the elbow.

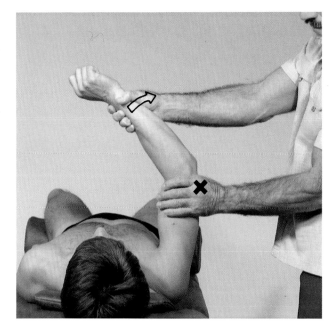

Fig. 34 a. Starting Position.

Procedure: Using this grip, T gradually and fully *extends* at P's elbow and simultaneously draws the forearm in the *ulnar* direction.

Stimulation of Antagonists: T retains grip . T then asks P to move further in the direction of stretching, and resists that movement to stimulate P's antagonists.

Note: This procedure may also be performed with P's forearm fully supinated.

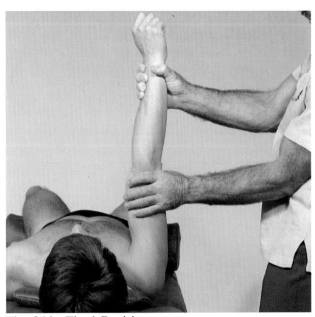

Fig. 34 b. Final Position.

3.3.3. Therapy for the **extensor carpi radialis longus.**

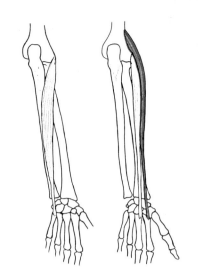

Starting Position: P: Supine; arm flexed approximately 90° and fully medially rotated; forearm flexed and fully pronated; wrist fully volar and ulnar flexed. T: Standing facing P's right side.

Grip: T's right hand grips wrist and proximal part of P's hand from the dorsal side while stabilizing P's wrist in full volar and *ulnar* flexion with the forearm fully pronated. T's left hand stabilizes P's upper arm at the dorsal side just proximal to the elbow.

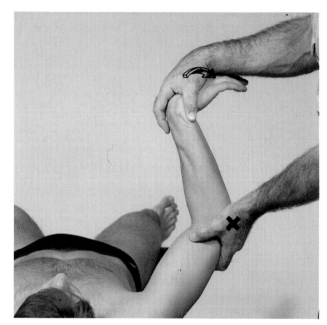

Fig. 35 a. Starting Position.

Procedure: Using this grip, T gradually and fully *extends* at P's elbow and simultaneously draws the forearm in the *ulnar* direction.

Stimulation of Antagonists: T reverses right-hand grip, moving right hand to volar side of P's right hand, and moving left hand to ventral side of P's elbow. T then asks P to move further in the direction of stretching, and resists that movement to stimulate P's antagonists.

Note: This technique and therapy is especially useful in treating epicondylitis.

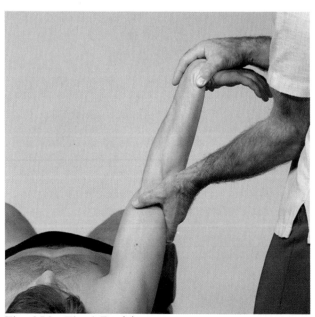

Fig. 35 b. Final Position.

54

3.3.4. Therapy for the **extensor carpi radialis brevis.**

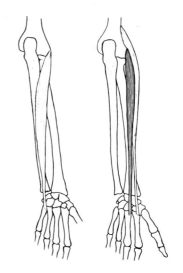

Starting Position: P: Supine; arm flexed approximately 90° and fully medially rotated; forearm flexed and fully pronated; hand in full volar flexion. T: Standing facing P's right side.

Grip: T's right hand grips the proximal part of P's hand at the dorsal side and stabilizes the hand in full volar flexion with the forearm fully pronated. T's left hand stabilizes P's upper arm at the dorsal side just proximal to the elbow.

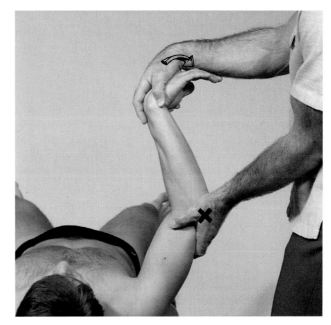

Fig. 36 a. Starting Position.

Procedure: Using this grip, T gradually and fully *extends* at P's elbow and simultaneously draws the forearm in the *ulnar* direction.

Stimulation of Antagonists: T reverses right-hand grip, moving right hand to volar side of P's right hand, and moving left hand to ventral side of elbow. T then asks P to move further in the direction of stretching, and resists that movement to stimulate P's antagonists.

Note: This technique and therapy is especially useful in treating epicondylitis.

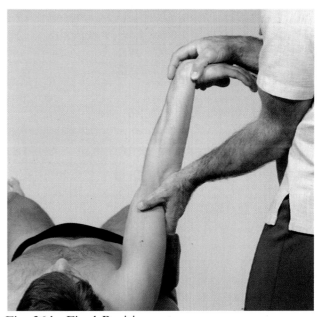

Fig. 36 b. Final Position.

55

3.3.5. Therapy for the **extensor digitorum communis**.

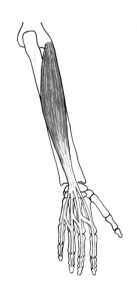

Starting Position: P: Supine; arm flexed approximately 90° and fully medially rotated; forearm flexed and fully pronated; hand fully volar flexed and fingers fully flexed at all joints. T: Standing facing P's right side.

Grip: T's right hand grips dorsal side of P's fingers so that full flexion is maintained at all finger joints. P's hand is held in full volar flexion, and the forearm is fully pronated. T's left hand stabilizes P's upper arm at the dorsal side just above the elbow.

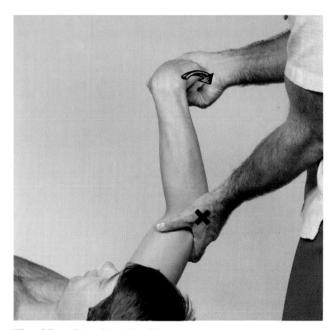

Fig. 37 a. Starting Position.

Procedure: Using this grip, T gradually and fully *extends* at P's elbow and simultaneously draws the forearm in the *ulnar* direction.

Stimulation of Antagonists: T retains right-hand grip, and reverses left-hand grip to ventral-medial side of P's elbow. T then asks P to move further in the direction of stretching, and resists that movement to stimulate P's antagonists.

Note: This technique and therapy is especially useful in treating epicondylitis.

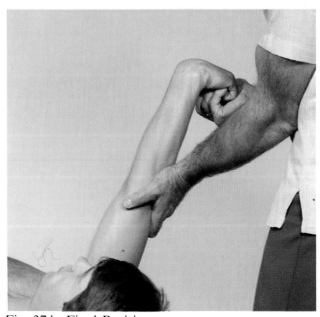

Fig. 37 b. Final Position.

3.3.6. Therapy for the **extensor indicis**.

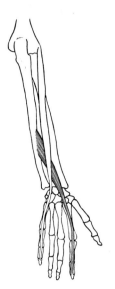

Starting Position: P: Supine; forearm flexed and fully pronated; index finger fully flexed at all the joints and in full radial flexion at the MCP joint. T: Standing at P's right side.

Grip: T's right hand grips dorsal side of P's index finger so that full flexion is maintained at all the joints while P's forearm is fully pronated. T's left hand grips just above P's wrist stabilizing P's forearm.

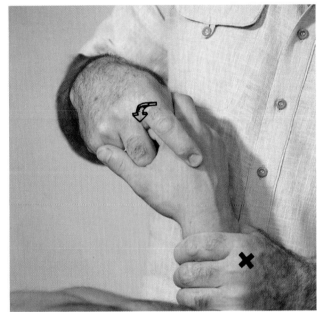

Fig. 38 a. Starting Position.

Procedure: Using this grip, T gradually and fully *volar flexes* at P's wrist.

Stimulation of Antagonists: T retains grip. T then asks P to move further in the direction of stretching, and resists that movement to stimulate P's antagonists.

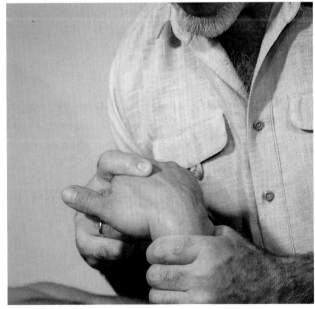

Fig. 38 b. Final Position.

3.3.7. Therapy for the **extensor digitorum communis.** *(Middle finger only).*

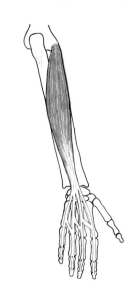

Starting Position: P: Supine; arm flexed approximately 90° and fully medially rotated; forearm flexed and fully pronated; hand fully volar flexed between radial and ulnar flexion; middle finger is in full flexion at all joints. T: Standing facing P's left side.

Grip: T's left hand grips dorsal side of P's middle finger so that full flexion is maintained at all the finger joints. T's right hand stabilizes P's upper arm just above the elbow.

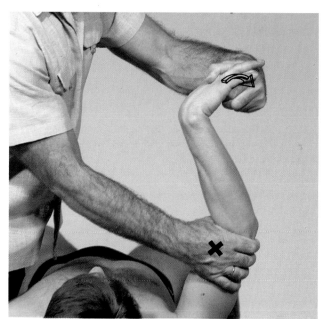

Fig. 39 a. Starting Position.

Procedure: Using this grip, T gradually and fully *extends* at P's elbow and simultaneously draws the forearm in an *ulnar* direction.

Stimulation of Antagonists: T retains grip. T then asks P to move further in the direction of stretching, and resists that movement to stimulate P's antagonists.

Note: This technique, and the previous one, 3.3.6, p. 57, are especially useful in treating epicondylitis.

Note: This technique and therapy is especially useful in treating epicondylitis.

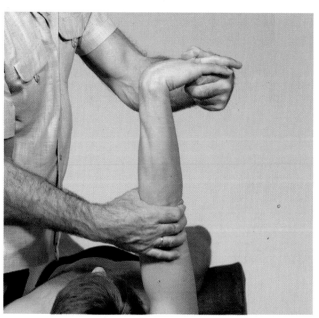

Fig. 39 b. Final Position.

3.3.8.   Therapy for the **extensor digiti minimi.**

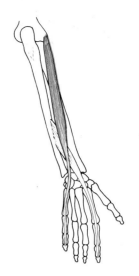

Starting Position: P: Supine; arm flexed approximately 90° and fully medially rotated; forearm flexed; hand in full volar and radial flexion; little finger fully flexed at all joints. T: Standing facing P's right side.

Grip: T's right hand grips dorsal side of P's little finger so that full flexion is maintained at all finger joints. T's left hand stabilizes P's upper arm just above the elbow.

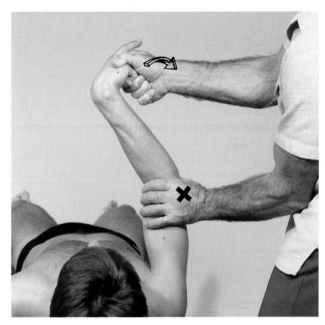

Fig. 40 a. Starting Position.

Procedure: Using this grip, T gradually and fully *extends* at P's elbow and simultaneously draws the forearm in the *ulnar* direction.

Stimulation of Antagonists: T retains grip. T then asks P to move further in the direction of stretching, and resists that movement to stimulate P's antagonists.

Note: This technique and therapy is especially useful in treating epicondylitis.

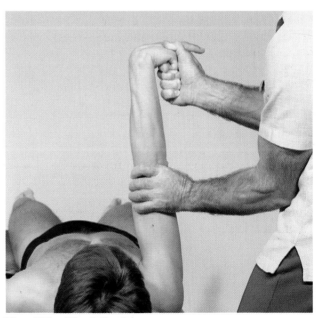

Fig. 40 b. Final Position.

3.3.9. Therapy for the **supinator**.

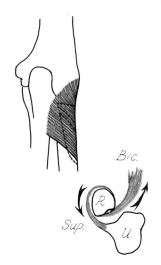

Starting Position: P: Supine; arm flexed approximately 90° and fully medially rotated; forearm flexed and fully pronated. T: Standing facing P's right side.

Grip: T's right hand grips dorsal side of P's forearm just above the wrist. T's left hand stabilizes P's upper arm at the dorsal side just above the elbow.

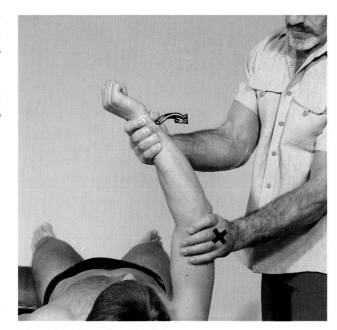

Fig. 41 a. Starting Position.

Procedure: Using this grip, T gradually and fully *extends* at P's elbow and simultaneously draws the forearm in the *ulnar* direction.

Stimulation of Antagonists: T retains grip. T then asks P to move further in the direction of stretching, and resists that movement to stimulate P's antagonists.

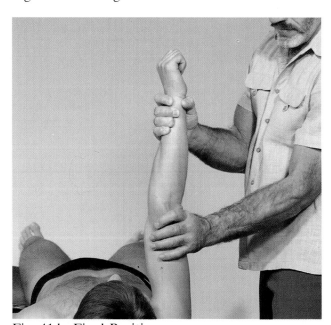

Fig. 41 b. Final Position.

3.3.10. Therapy for the **extensor carpi ulnaris.**

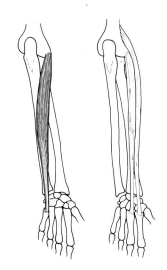

Starting Position: P: Supine; arm flexed approximately 90° and fully medially rotated; forearm pronated; hand in full volar and radial flexion. T: Standing facing P's right side.

Grip: T's right hand grips wrist and proximal part of P's hand from the dorsal side. T's left hand stabilizes P's upper arm at the dorsal side just above the elbow.

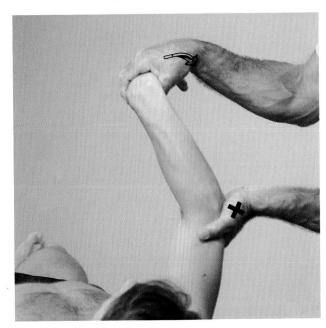

Fig. 42 a. Starting Position.

Procedure: Using this grip, T gradually and fully *extends* at P's elbow and simultaneously draws the forearm in the *ulnar* direction.

Stimulation of Antagonists: T retains grip. T then asks P to move further in the direction of stretching, and resists that movement to stimulate P's antagonists.

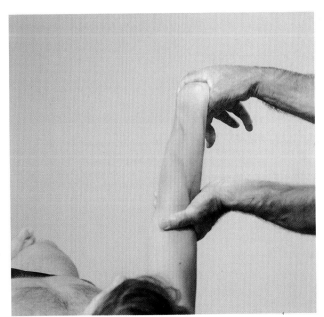

Fig. 42 b. Final Position.

3.3.11. Therapy for the **flexor carpi ulnaris**.

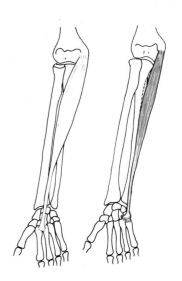

Starting Position: P: Supine; arm flexed approximately 90° and fully laterally rotated; forearm flexed and fully supinated; hand in full dorsal and radial flexion. T: standing facing P's right side.

Grip: T's right hand grips the proximal part of P's palm and fingers, holding the fingers fully flexed. T's left hand stabilizes P's elbow at the dorsal side.

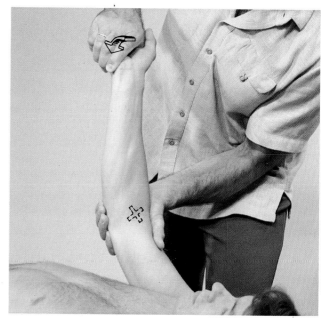

Fig. 43 a. Starting Position.

Procedure: Using this grip, T gradually and fully *extends* at P's elbow and simultaneously pushes the forearm in the *ulnar* direction.

Stimulation of Antagonists: T retains grip. T then asks P to move further in the direction of stretching, and resists that movement to stimulate P's antagonists.

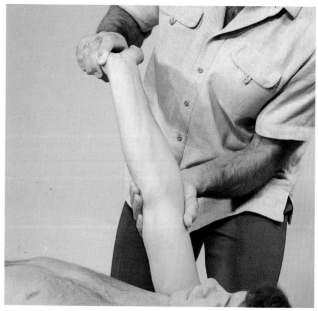

Fig. 43 b. Final Position.

3.3.12. Therapy for the **flexor carpi radialis.**

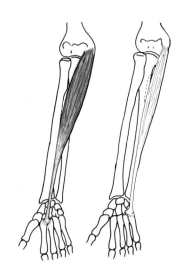

Starting Position: P: Supine; arm flexed approximately 90° and fully laterally rotated; forearm flexed and fully supinated; hand in full dorsal and ulnar flexion. T: Standing facing P's right side.

Grip: T's right hand grips the radial-volar side of the proximal part of P's hand so MCP joints are free to flex. T's left hand stabilizes P's upper arm at the dorsal side at the elbow.

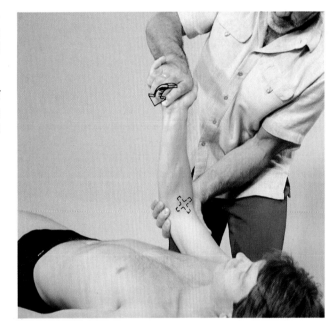

Fig. 44 a. Starting Position.

Procedure: Using this grip, T gradually and fully *extends* at P's elbow and simultaneously pushes on the forearm in the *ulnar* direction.

Stimulation of Antagonists: T retains grip. T then asks P to move further in the direction of stretching, and resists that movement to stimulate P's antagonists.

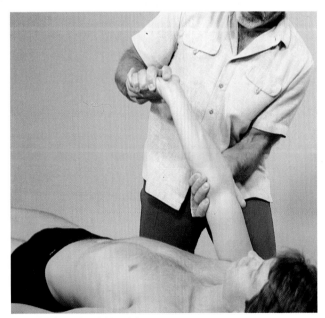

Fig. 44 b. Final Position.

3.3.13. Therapy for the **flexor digitorum superficialis.**

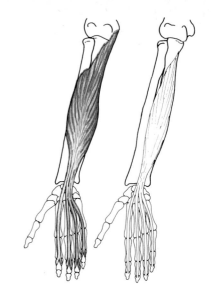

Starting Position: P: Supine: arm abducted and fully laterally rotated; forearm flexed and fully supinated; hand in full dorsal flexion; fingers fully extended at the PIP and MCP joints. T: Sitting on couch, back against P's right side.

Grip: T's left hand grips P's palm and fingers so the DIP joints are free to flex. T's right hand stabilizes P's upper arm at the medial side just above the elbow.

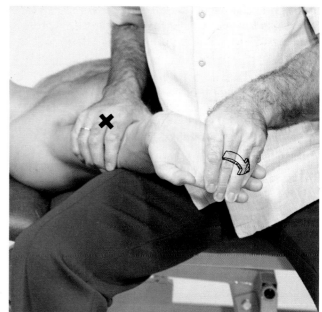

Fig. 45 a. Starting Position.

Procedure: Using this grip, T gradually and fully *extends* at P's elbow and simultaneously pulls on the forearm in the *ulnar* direction.

Stimulation of Antagonists: T retains grip. T then asks P to move further in the direction of stretching, and resists that movement to stimulate P's antagonists.

Note: The **palmaris longus** is also stretched in this procedure.

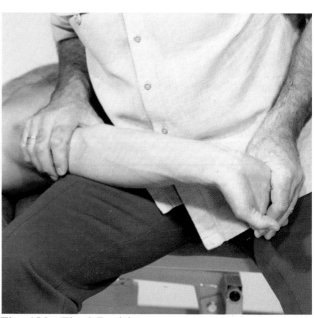

Fig. 45 b. Final Position.

3.3.14. Therapy for the **pronator teres, humeral head.**

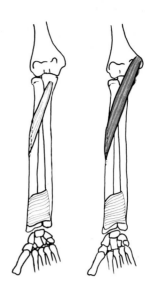

Starting Position: P: Supine; arm flexed approximately 90° and fully laterally rotated; forearm flexed and fully supinated. T: Sitting on couch, back against P's right side.

Grip: T's left hand grips dorsal side of P's forearm just above the wrist. T's right hand stabilizes P's upper arm at the ventral side just above the elbow.

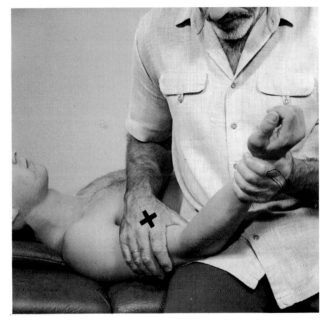

Fig. 46 a. Starting Position.

Procedure: Using this grip, T gradually and fully *extends* at P's elbow and simultaneously draws the forearm maximally in the *ulnar* direction.

Stimulation of Antagonists: T retains grip. T then asks P to move further in the direction of stretching, and resists that movement to stimulate P's antagonists.

Note: The **pronator teres, ulnar head** and the **pronator quadratus** are also stretched in this procedure.

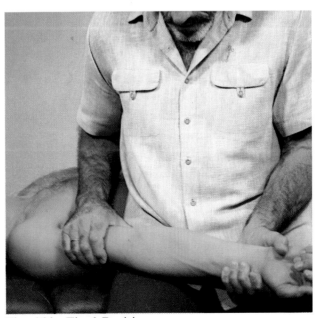

Fig. 46 b. Final Position.

65

3.3.15. Therapy for the **pronator teres, ulnar head** and the **pronator quadratus.**

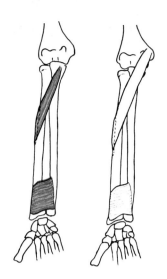

Starting Position: P: Supine; elbow flexed approximately 90°.
T: Sitting on couch, right side against P's right side.

Grip: T's left hand grips dorsal side of P's forearm just above the wrist. T's right hand stabilizes P's upper arm at the medial side just above the elbow.

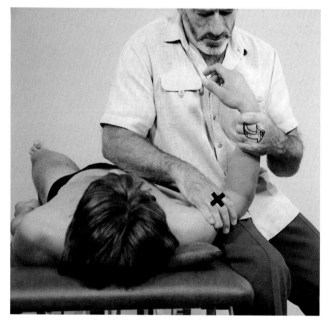

Fig. 47 a. Starting Position.

Procedure: Using this grip, T gradually and maximally *supinates* P's forearm.

Stimulation of Antagonists: T retains grip. T then asks P to move further in the direction of stretching, and resists that movement to stimulate P's antagonists.

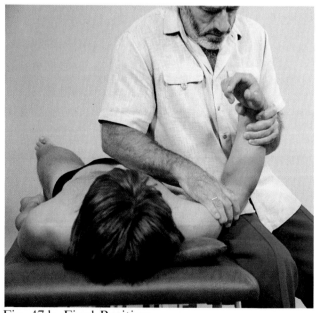

Fig. 47 b. Final Position.

3.3.16.   Therapy for the **palmaris longus.**

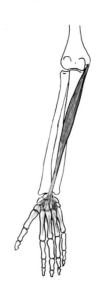

Starting Position: P: Supine; shoulder abducted and fully laterally rotated; elbow flexed and forearm fully supinated; wrist in full dorsal flexion with MCP joints fully extended. T: Sitting, back against P's right side.

Grip: T's left hand grips the proximal part of P's hand from the ulnar-volar side down to the MCP joints. T's right hand stabilizes P's upper arm at the medial side just above the elbow.

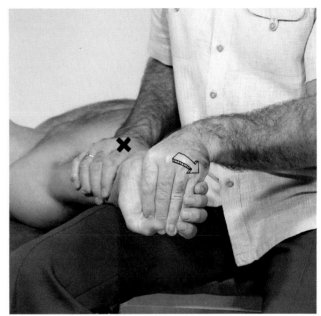

Fig. 48 a. Starting Position.

Procedure: Using this grip, T gradually and fully *extends* at P's elbow and simultaneously pulls on the forearm in the *ulnar* direction.

Stimulation of Antagonists: T retains grip. T then asks P to move further in the direction of stretching, and resists that movement to stimulate P's antagonists.

Note: To *maximally* stretch the **palmaris longus** in this procedure, it may be necessary to fully extend P's fingers.

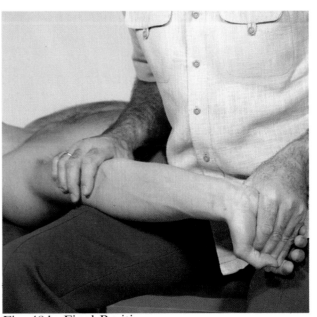

Fig. 48 b. Final Position.

4   THE WRIST

4.1   THERAPY GUIDE

The muscles which may restrict movement at the wrist are listed in Table 4-1, along with the applicable therapies, indexed by manual section number and page. Muscle actions are listed in Table 4-2. The various restrictions possible are listed in Movement Restriction Table 10.4 (p. 168).

Table 4-1. Restrictions at the wrist

SECTION	MOVEMENT RESTRICTED	MUSCLES WHICH MAY RESTRICT MOTION	THERAPY	Number	Page
4.2.	*Volar flexion*	Extensor digitorum communis		3.3.5, 3.3.7	56, 58
		Extensor pollicis longus		4.2.1	70
		Extensor indicis		3.3.6	57
		Extensor digiti minimi		3.3.8	59
		Extensor carpi radialis longus		3.3.3	54
		Extensor carpi radialis brevis		3.3.4	55
		Extensor carpi ulnaris		3.3.10	61
4.3	*dorsal flexion*	Palmaris longus		3.3.16	67
		Flexor carpi ulnaris		3.3.11	62
		Flexor digitorum superficialis		3.3.13	64
		Flexor digitorum profundus		4.3.1	71
		Flexor pollicis longus		4.3.2	72
4.4	*Radial flexion*	Flexor carpi ulnaris		3.3.11, 4.4.1	62, 73
		Extensor carpi ulnaris		3.3.10, 4.4.1	61, 73
4.5	*Ulnar flexion*	Abductor pollicis longus		4.5.1	74
		Extensor pollicis brevis		4.5.2	75
		Flexor carpi radialis		3.3.10	61
		Extensor carpi radialis longus		3.3.3	54

Table 4-2. Actions of muscles which may restrict movement at the wrist.

MUSCLE	ACTION
Extensor digitorum communis	Extends fingers. Flexes at elbow. Supinates forearm. Dorsal flexes at wrist.
Extensor pollicis longus	Extends thumb. Supinates forearm. Dorsal and radial flexes at wrist.
Extensor pollicis brevis	Extends thumb at CMC- and MCP-joints (and often IP-joint). Radial flexes at wrist. Volar or dorsal flexes at wrist (depending on position of hand). Supinates forearm.
Extensor indicis	Extends and ulnar deviates index finger. Supinates forearm. Dorsal flexes at wrist.
Extensor digiti minimi	Extends little finger. Flexes at elbow. Dorsal and ulnar flexes at wrist.
Extensor carpi radialis longus and brevis	Flex at elbow. Supinate forearm. Dorsal and radial flex at wrist.
Extensor carpi ulnaris	Dorsal and ulnar flexes at wrist. Flexes at elbow. Supinates forearm.
Palmaris longus	Flexes at elbow. Pronates forearm. Volar flexes at wrist.
Flexor carpi ulnaris	Flexes at elbow. Pronates forearm. Volar and ulnar flexes at wrist.
Flexor carpi radialis	Flexes at elbow. Pronates forearm. Volar and radial flexes at wrist.
Flexor digitorum super-ficialis	Flexes fingers (including at PIP joints). Flexes at elbow. Volar flexes at wrist.
Flexor digitorum pro-fundus	Flexes all finger joints except thumb. Volar flexes at wrist.
Flexor pollicis longus	Opposes and flexes thumb. Volar flexes at wrist. May pronate forearm. Flexes at elbow (rarely).
Abductor pollicis longus	Abducts thumb. Radial and volar flexes at wrist. Supinates forearm.

NOTES: 1. Actions described in terms most relevant to manual therapy. Cross-reference to terms often used in anatomy texts:

Ulnar flexion (towards ulna), corresponds to adduction (usually of hand)
Radial flexion (towards radius), corresponds to abduction (usually of hand)
Volar flexion (towards palm), corresponds to flexion of hand
dorsal flexion (towards back of hand), corresponds to extension of hand

2. Finger joint abbreviations: CCM – Carpo-metacarpal, IP – Interphalangeal, MCP – Metacarpo-phalangeal, PIP – Proximal – interphalangeal.

4.2.1.   Therapy for the **extensor pollicis longus.**

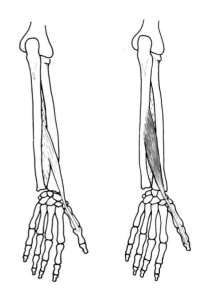

Starting Position: P: Supine; upper arm and elbow rest on couch; elbow at approximately 90° flexion; forearm fully pronated; wrist in neutral position with thumb in full flexion and opposition. T: Standing facing P's right side.

Grip: T's left hand grips radial side of P's thumb and stabilizes it in full flexion and opposition against P's palm. T's right hand stabilizes P's forearm at the ulnar side.

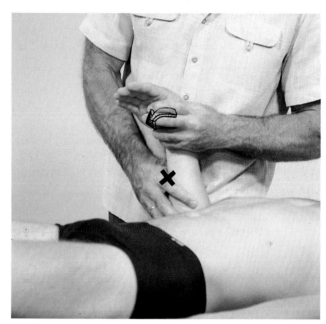

Fig. 49 a. Starting Position.

Procedure: Using this grip, T gradually and fully *volar* and *ulnar flexes* at P's wrist while simultaneously pronating P's forearm.

Stimulation of Antagonists: T retains grip. T then asks P to move further in the direction of stretching, and resists that movement to stimulate P's antagonists.

Note: The **extensor pollicis brevis** is also stretched in this procedure.

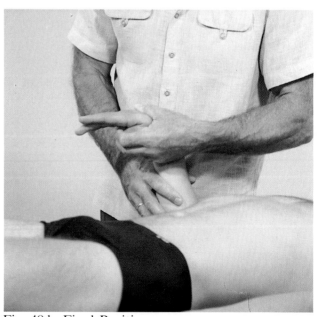

Fig. 49 b. Final Position.

70

4.3.1. Therapy for the **flexor digitorum profundus.**

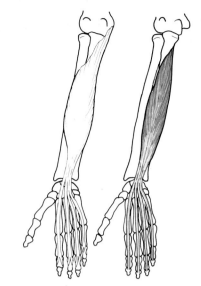

Starting Position: P: Supine; elbow flexed 90° and forearm fully supinated; wrist in neutral position with all finger joints, including the MCP joints, fully extended. T: Sitting on couch, back against P's right side.

Grip: T's left hand grips volar sides of P's fingers and fully extends all joints, including the MCP joints. (Note that P's wrist remains in the neutral position or slightly volar flexed). T's right hand stabilizes P's forearm at the medial side just above the wrist.

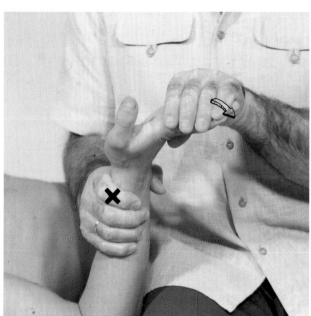

Fig. 50 a. Starting Position.

Procedure: Using this grip, T gradually and fully *dorsal flexes* at P's wrist.

Stimulation of Antagonists: T retains grip. T then asks P to move further in the direction of stretching, and resists that movement to stimulate P's antagonists.

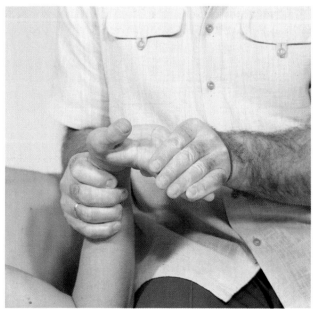

Fig. 50 b. Final Position.

4.3.2. Therapy for the **flexor pollicis longus.**

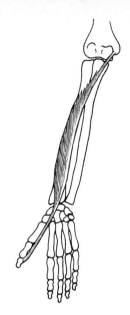

Starting Position: P: Supine; upper arm and elbow resting against the couch or against T's abdomen or thigh; elbow flexed approximately 90° and forearm fully supinated; wrist in neutral position with thumb fully extended.
T: Standing with right side against P.

Grip: T's left hand grips P's entire thumb from the volar side and extends it maximally. T's right hand holds P's hand from the ulnar/volar aspect, index and middle finger around radial side of hand.

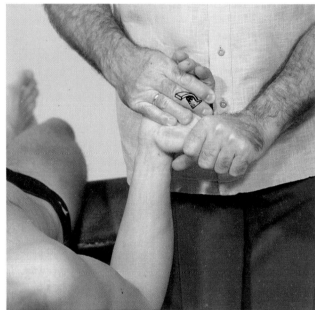

Fig. 51 a. Starting Position.

Procedure: Using this grip, T gradually and fully supinates forearm and *dorsal flexes* at P's wrist.

Stimulation of Antagonists: T retains grip. T then asks P to move further in the direction of stretching, and resists that movement to stimulate P's antagonists.

Note: In anomalous cases where the **flexor pollicis longus** also originates from the medial epicondyle of the humerus, it will be necessary to fully extend P's elbow to attain maximal stretching. Extension of P's thumb is more restricted than when the elbow is flexed.

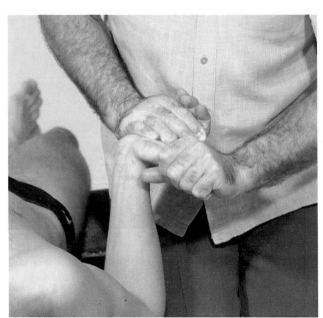

Fig. 51 b. Final Position.

72

4.4.1. Therapy for the **flexor carpi ulnaris** and the **extensor carpi ulnaris**.

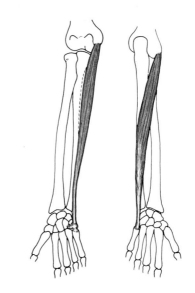

Starting Position: P: Supine or sitting; right arm extended, ulnar side resting on couch; wrist in neutral position. T: Standing, left side against P.

Grip: T's right hand grips P's hand, palm-to-palm ("handshake" grip) with radial side of index finger touching the pisiform bone. T's left hand stabilizes P's extended arm against couch.

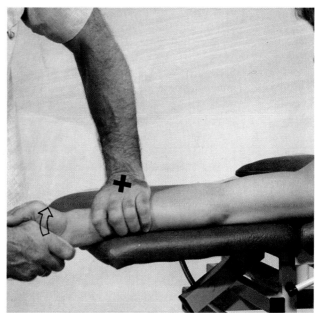

Fig. 52 a. Starting Position.

Procedure: Using this grip, T gradually and fully *radial flexes* at P's wrist.

Stimulation of Antagonists: T retains grip. T then asks P to move further in the direction of stretching, and resists that movement to stimulate P's antagonists.

Notes: Insufficient ulnar glide may constrain the treatment's radial flexing. Therefore, during treatment T should feel for free ulnar glide. If ulnar glide is restricted, T should mobilize wrist to restore ulnar glide.

Radial flexion may also be restricted in combination with dorsal or volar flexion. If so, procedure should accordingly be followed with wrist dorsally or volar flexed.

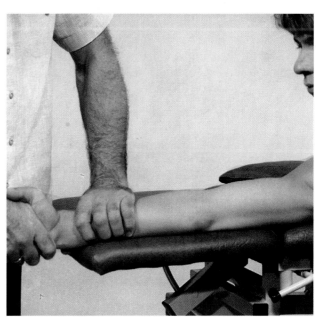

Fig. 52 b. Final Position.

73

4.5.1. Therapy for the **abductor pollicis longus.**

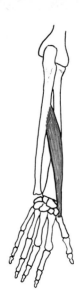

Starting Position: P: Supine or sitting; elbow flexed approximately 90°; forearm fully pronated; wrist in neutral position. T: Standing, right side against P.

Grip: T places thenar eminence of right hand over P's first metacarpal bone (from dorsal side) with his fingers gripping the ulnar border of P's hand (from volar side). T's left hand stabilizes P's forearm just above the wrist.

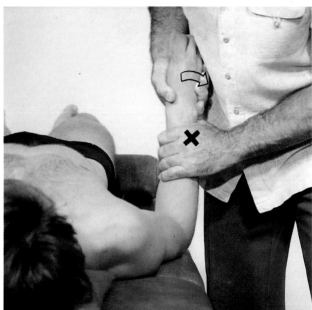

Fig. 53 a. Starting Position.

Procedure: Using this grip, T gradually and maximally *ulnar flexes* at P's wrist.

Stimulation of Antagonists: T retains grip. T then asks P to move further in the direction of stretching, and resists that movement to stimulate P's antagonists.

Note: For maximal stretching of the **abductor pollicis longus** in this procedure, T may simultaneously fully dorsally flex at P's wrist.

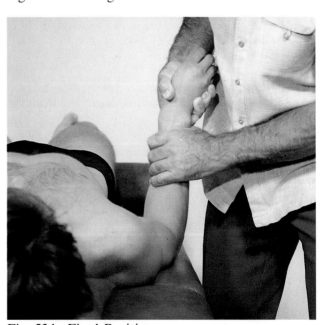

Fig. 53 b. Final Position.

4.5.2. Therapy for the **extensor pollicis brevis.**

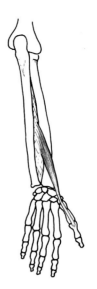

Starting Position: P: Supine or sitting; elbow at approximately 90° flexion; forearm fully pronated with wrist in neutral position; thumb against palm, in full opposition and flexion at all joints. T: Standing facing P's right side.

Grip: T's right hand grips P's hand and thumb from the volar side, palm-to-palm, and holds P's thumb fully opposed and flexed in all joints. T's left hand stabilizes P's forearm just above the wrist.

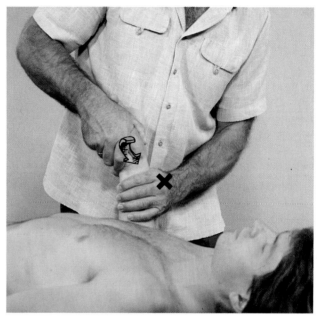

Fig. 54 a. Starting Position.

Procedure: Using this grip, T gradually and maximally *ulnar* and *dorsal flexes* at P's wrist while fully pronating P's forearm.

Stimulation of Antagonists: T retains grip. T then asks P to move further in the direction of stretching, and resists that movement to stimulate P's antagonists.

Note: If the position of greatest restriction is attained with the wrist in volar flexion, then it is necessary to treat in that position.

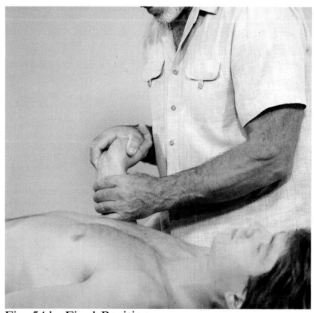

Fig. 54 b. Final Position.

5 THE FINGERS

5.1 THERAPY GUIDE

The muscles which may restrict movements of the fingers are listed in Table 5-1, along with the applicable therapies, indexed by manual section number and page. Muscle actions are listed in Table 5-2.
The various restrictions possible are listed in Movement Restriction Tables 10.5, 10.6 and 10.7 (pp. 169-171).

TABLE 5.1   Restrictions at the fingers

SECTION	MOVEMENT RESTRICTED	RESTRICTING MUSCLE(S)	THERAPY	Number	Page
5.2	*Flexion*	Extensor digitorum communis		3.3.5, 3.3.7	56, 58
		Extensor indicis		3.3.6	57
		Extensor digiti minimi		3.3.8	59
		Interossei dorsales[1]		5.2.1	79
		Interossei palmares[1]		5.2.2	80
		Lumbricales[1]		5.2.3	81
5.3	*Extension*	Flexor pollicis brevis		5.3.1	82
		Flexor pollicis longus		4.3.2	72
		Flexor digitorum superficialis		3.3.13	64
		Flexor digitorum profundus		4.3.1	71
		Interossei dorsales[2]		5.2.1	79
		Interossei palmares[2]		5.2.2	80
		Lumbricales[2]		5.2.3	81
		Flexor digiti minimi brevis		5.2.2	80
5.4	*Abduction of thumb*	Adductor pollicis and/or Interosseus palmaris I		5.4.1	83
5.5	*Adduction of thumb*	Abductor pollicis longus		4.5.1	74
		Abductor pollicis brevis		5.5.1	84
5.6	*Opposition of thumb*	Extensor pollicis longus and brevis, Interosseus palmaris I and		5.6.1	85
				4.2.1	70
		Abductor pollicis longus,		4.5.2	75
		together		5.2.3	80, 83
		Individually		4.5.1	74
5.7	*Reposition of thumb*	Flexor pollicis longus		4.3.2	72
		Flexor pollicis brevis		5.3.1	82
		Opponens pollicis and/or Adductor pollicis, transverse head		5.7.1	86
5.8	*Opposition of little finger*	Abductor digiti minimi		5.8.1	87
		Extensor digiti minimi		3.3.8	59
5.9	*Reposition of little finger*	Flexor digiti minimi brevis		5.2.2	80
		Opponens digiti minimi		5.9.1	88

NOTES: 1:   Restricts only at DIP and PIP joints; 2: Restricts only at MCP joints.

TABLE 5.2 Actions of muscles which may restrict movements at the fingers

MUSCLE	ACTION
Muscles of the forearm	
Extensor digitorum communis	Extends fingers. Flexes at elbow. Supinates forearm. Dorsal flexes at wrist.
Extensor indicis	Extends and ulnar deviates index finger. Supinates forearm. Dorsal flexes at wrist.
Extensor digiti minimi	Extends little finger. Flexes at elbow. Dorsal and ulnar flexes at wrist.
Flexor pollicis longus	Opposes and flexes thumb. Volar flexes at wrist. May pronate forearm. Flexes at elbow (rarely).
Flexor digitorum superficialis	Flexes fingers (including at PIP joints). Flexes at elbow. Volar flexes at wrist.
Flexor digitorum profundus	Flexes all finger joints except thumb. Volar flexes at wrist.
Abductor pollicis longus	Abducts thumb. Radial and volar flexes at wrist. Supinates forearm.
Extensor pollicis longus	Extends thumb. Supinates forearm. Dorsal and radial flexes at wrist.
Extensor pollicis brevis	Extends thumb at CMC and MCP joints (and often at IP joint). Radial flexes at wrist. Volar or dorsal flexes at wrist (depending on position of hand). Supinates forearm.
Muscles of the hand	
Interossei dorsales[1]	Flex at MCP joints. Extend at DIP and PIP joints. Abduct fingers away from axial line through middle finger.
Interossei palmares[1]	Flex at MCP joints. Extend at DIP and PIP joints. Adduct fingers toward axial line through middle finger.
Lumbricales[1]	Flex at MCP joints. Extend at DIP and PIP joints.
Flexor digiti minimi brevis	Flexes at MCP joint of little finger.
Flexor pollicis brevis	Flexes at MCP joint and assists opposition of thumb.
Adductor pollicis	Adducts thumb. Transverse head also opposes thumb.
Abductor pollicis brevis	Abducts thumb at MCP and CMC joints.
Opponens pollicis	Opposes and adducts thumb
Opponens digiti minimi	Flexes little finger at CMC joint; opposes little finger.
Abductor digiti minimi	Abducts and flexes at MCP joint of little finger

NOTES: 1. The interossei dorsales, interossei palmares, and/or lumbricales may restrict finger flexion only at the DIP/and PIP joints, and may restrict finger extension only at the MCP joints.
  2. Actions described in terms most relevant to manual therapy. Cross reference to terms often used in anatomy texts:

Ulnar flexion:	towards ulna, corresponds to adduction (usually of hand)
Radial flexion:	towards radius, corresponds to abduction (usually of hand)
Volar flexion:	towards palm, corresponds to flexion of hand
Dorsal flexion:	towards back of hand, corresponds to extension of hand

  3. Finger joint abbreviations:

CMC Carpo-metacarpal
IP   Interphalangeal
MCP Metacarpo-phalangeal
PIP Proximal-interphalangeal

5.2.1. Therapy for the **interossei dorsales**. (Stretching of **interosseus dorsalis I** shown)

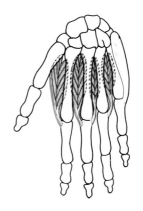

Starting position: P: Supine or sitting; elbow flexed approximately 90° and supported against the couch; wrist in neutral position; MCP joint slightly flexed and DIP and PIP joints in full flexion. T: Standing facing P's right side.

Grip: T grips P's index finger with right hand, thumb on dorsal side, and holds the DIP and PIP joints fully flexed. T's left hand stabilizes P's wrist and hand at the dorsal side.

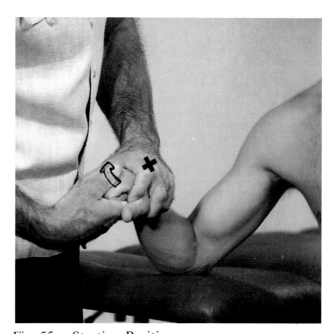

Fig. 55 a. Starting Position.

Procedure: Using this grip, T gradually and fully *extends* and *adducts* (in the ulnar direction) at the MCP joint of P's index finger.

Stimulation of Antagonists: T retains grip. T then asks P to move further in the direction of stretching, and resists that movement to stimulate P's antagonists.

Notes: T should apply slight traction to assure good glide at the MCP joint. If dorsal glide at the MCP joint is painful and/or restricted, T should apply slight traction while assuring dorsal glide.

Same grip and procedure for other three fingers, with following exceptions:

Finger	Interosseus dorsalis	Additional grip procedure
Middle	II	Middle finger abducted in *ulnar* direction
Ring	III	Middle finger adducted in *radial* direction
Little	IV	Ring finger adducted in *radial* direction

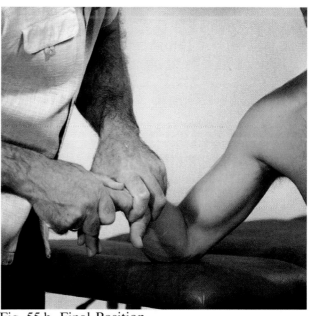

Fig. 55 b. Final Position.

5.2.2. Therapy for the **interossei palmares**. (Stretching of **interosseus palmaris IV** shown.)

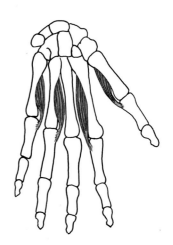

Starting Position: P: Supine or sitting; elbow flexed approximately 90°; wrist in neutral position; all joints of little finger fully flexed. T: Standing, left side against P.

Grip: T's right hand grips P's little finger (or all P's fingers simultaneously) and holds the DIP, PIP and MCP joints fully flexed. T's left hand stabilizes P's wrist.

Procedure: Using this grip, T gradually and fully *extends* and *abducts* (in the ulnar direction) at the MCP joint of P's little finger.

Stimulation of Antagonists: T retains grip. T then asks P to move further in the direction of stretching, and resists that movement to stimulate P's antagonists.

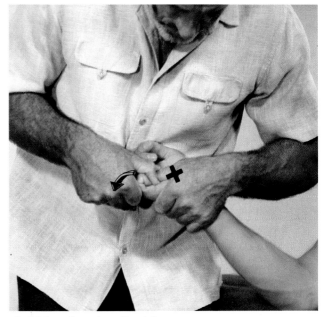

Fig. 56 a. Starting Position.

Notes: While extending the MCP joints during the procedure, T applies traction with dorsal gliding. If the joints are painful it is advisable to stretch only one muscle at a time.

The **flexor digiti minimi brevis** is also stretched in this procedure.

Same grip and procedure for the other three fingers, with following exceptions.

Finger	Interosseus palmaris	Additional grip procedure
Thumb	I	Thumb finger abducted in *radial direction*
Index	II	Index finger abducted in *radial* direction
Ring	III	Ring finger abducted in *ulnar* direktion

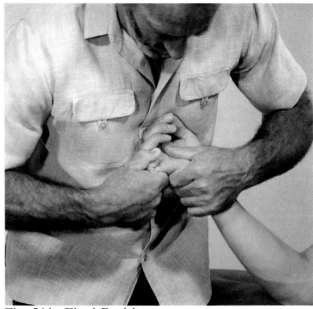

Fig. 56 b. Final Position.

5.2.3.   Therapy for the **lumbricales.**

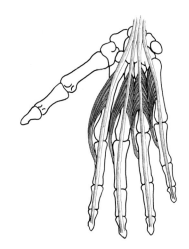

Starting Position: P: Supine or sitting; elbow flexed approximately 90°; forearm fully supinated; wrist in neutral position; MCP joints fully extended; DIP and PIP joints fully flexed. T: Standing, left side against P's right side.

Grip: T's right hand grips all of P's fingers, holding them fully extended at the MCP joints and fully flexed at the DIP and PIP joints. T's left hand stabilizes P's forearm just above the wrist.

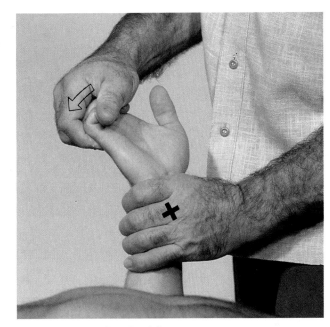

Fig. 57 a. Starting Position.

Procedure: Using this grip, T gradually and fully *dorsally flexes* at P's wrist.

Stimulation of Antagonists: T retains grip. T then asks P to move further in the direction of stretching, and resists that movement to stimulate P's antagonists.

Notes: P's flexed elbow can be supported against the couch with T's left hand gripping P's hand at the volar side. This enables T to use both hands to obtain maximal stretching.

Stretching the **lumbricales** individually, one at a time, is most effective.

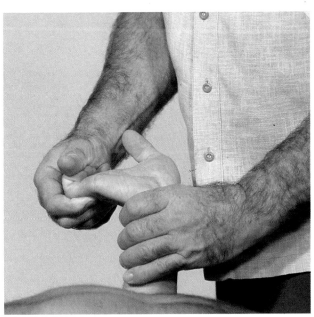

Fig. 57 b. Final Position.

5.3.1. Therapy for the **flexor pollicis brevis.**

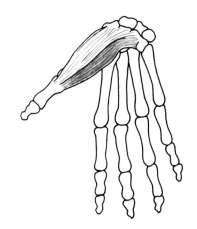

Starting Position: P: Supine or sitting; elbow flexed approximately 90° and steadied against the couch; forearm fully supinated; wrist in neutral position; thumb extended. T: Standing facing P.

Grip: T's left hand grips the proximal phalanx of P's thumb. T's right hand stabilizes P's hand from the volar aspect.

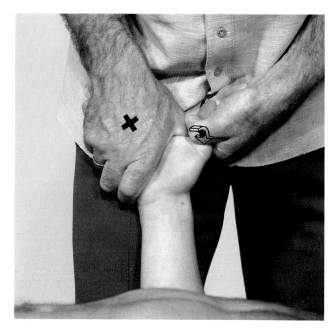

Fig. 58 a. Starting Position.

Procedure: Using this grip, T gradually and fully *extends* P's thumb.

Stimulation of Antagonists: T retains grip. T then asks P to move further in the direction of stretching, and resists that movement to stimulate P's antagonists.

Notes: During the procedure, it may also be necessary to stretch by fully *dorsally flexing* at P's wrist when extension is most restricted in this position.

The **interosseus palmaris I** is also stretched in this procedure.

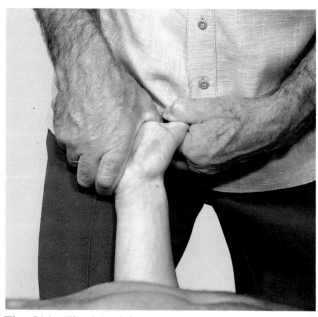

Fig. 58 b. Final Position.

5.4.1. Therapy for the **adductor pollicis** and the **interosseus palmaris I.**

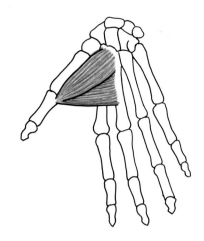

Starting Position: P: Supine or sitting; elbow flexed approximately 90° and steadied against the couch; wrist in neutral position. T: Standing facing P's right side.

Grip: T's right hand grips proximal phalanx of the thumb and the base of the first metacarpal bone of P's hand. T's left hand stabilizes P's hand from the dorsal/radial aspect with T's thumb against P's palm.

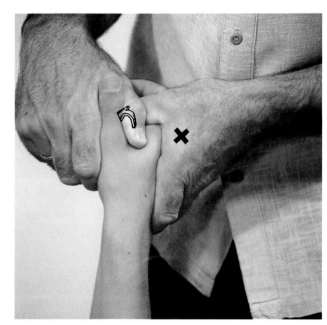

Fig. 59 a. Starting Position.

Procedure: Using this grip, T gradually and fully *abducts* P's thumb and simultaneously applies traction.

Stimulation of Antagonists: T retains grip. T then asks P to move further in the direction of stretching, and resists that movement to stimulate P's antagonists.

Note: For maximal stretching, P's thumb should also be medially rotated.

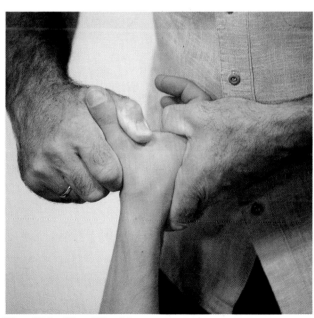

Fig. 59 b. Final Position.

5.5.1.   Therapy for the **abductor pollicis brevis.**

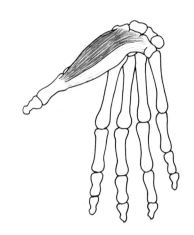

Starting Position: P: Supine or sitting; elbow flexed approximately 90° and steadied against the couch; forearm fully pronated with wrist in full dorsal flexion; thumb fully extended at MCP joint. T: Standing facing P's right side.

Grip: T's right hand grips the first metacarpal bone and the proximal phalanx of P's thumb from the volar side, with thenar eminence stabilizing P's first metacarpal bone. T's left hand stabilizes P's hand dorsally and holds P's wrist fully dorsal and ulnar flexed.

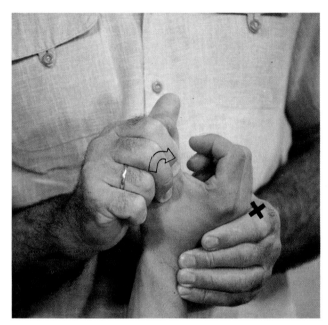

Fig. 60 a. Starting Position.

Procedure: Using this grip, T applies traction and gradually and fully *adducts* P's thumb.

Stimulation of Antagonists: T retains grip. T then asks P to move further in the direction of stretching, and resists that movement to stimulate P's antagonists.

Note: To attain *maximal* stretching, it may be necessary to position P's arm with the elbow extended and the forearm fully supinated.

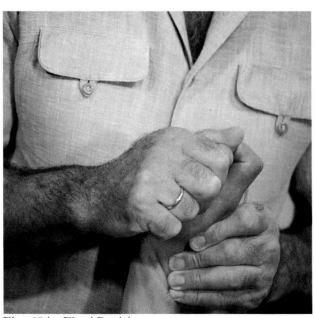

Fig. 60 b. Final Position.

5.6.1. Therapy for the **extensor pollicis longus and brevis**, the **interosseus palmaris I**, and the **abductor pollicis longus**.

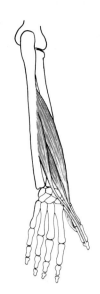

Starting Position: P: Supine or sitting; ulnar side of forearm and hand steadied against couch; forearm fully pronated with wrist in neutral position.
T: Standing, left side against P's right side.

Grip: T's left hand grips P's thumb with T's thenar eminence against the dorsal side of P's first metacarpal bone. T's right hand stabilizes P's hand from the ulnar-dorsal side.

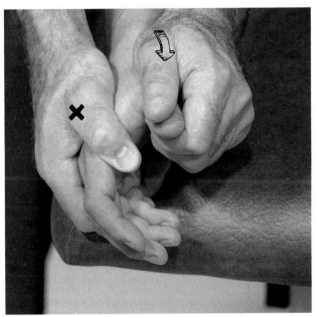

Fig. 61 a. Starting Position.

Procedure: Using this grip, T gradually and fully *opposes* P's thumb while simultaneously applying traction to the CMC joint of the thumb.

Stimulation of Antagonists: T retains grip. T then asks P to move further in the direction of stretching, and resists that movement to stimulate P's antagonists.

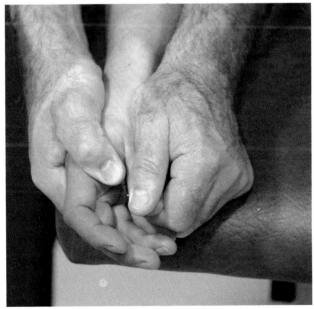

Fig. 61 b. Final Position.

5.7.1. Therapy for the **opponens pollicis and the adductor pollicis, transverse head.**

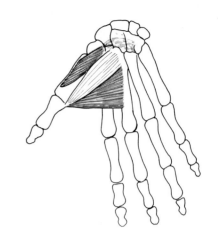

Starting Position: P: Supine or sitting; elbow flexed approximately 90° and steadied against the couch; wrist in neutral position; thumb extended. T: Standing facing P's right side.

Grip: T's left hand grips the proximal phalanx of P's thumb and first metacarpal bone. T's right hand stabilizes P's hand at the volar-radial side.

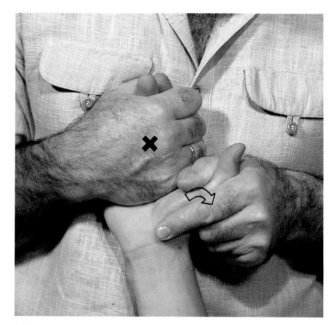

Fig. 62 a. Starting Position.

Procedure: Using this grip, T gradually and fully *reposes* P's thumb and simultaneously applies traction to the CMC joint of the thumb.

Stimulation of Antagonists: T retains grip. T then asks P to move further in the direction of stretching, and resists that movement to stimulate P's antagonists.

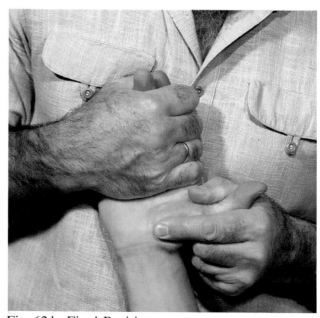

Fig. 62 b. Final Position.

5.8.1. Therapy for the **abductor digiti minimi.**

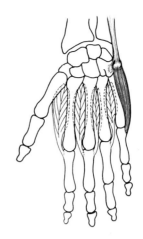

Starting Position: P: Supine or sitting; elbow extended and forearm fully supinated; wrist in full dorsal and radial flexion; all fingers fully flexed. T: Standing, back against P.

Grip: T's left hand grips P's flexed little finger, with index finger over P's distal phalanx and his thumb close to P's MCP joint on the dorsal side. T's right hand stabilizes P's thumb and the rest of P's fingers at the radial side.

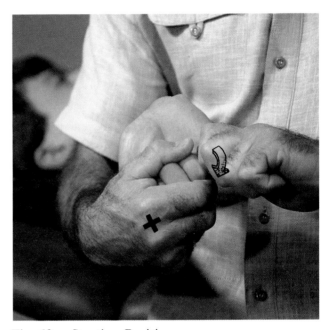

Fig. 63 a. Starting Position.

Procedure: Using this grip, T gradually and fully *extends* and *adducts* (in the radial direction) at the MCP joint of P's little finger.

Stimulation of Antagonists: T retains grip. T then asks P to move further in the direction of stretching, and resists that movement to stimulate P's antagonists.

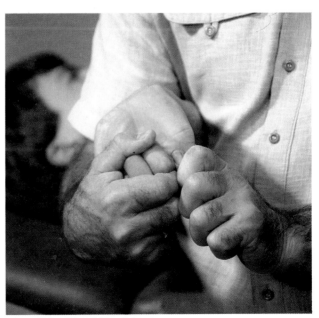

Fig. 63 b. Final Position.

5.9.1. Therapy for the **opponens digiti minimi.**

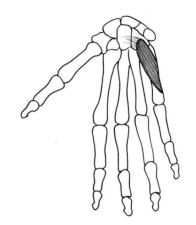

Starting Position: P: Supine or sitting; elbow flexed approximately 90°; forearm fully pronated with wrist fully dorsally flexed; fingers flexed. T: Standing, left side against P.

Grip: T's right hand grips P's hypothenar eminence, thumb over volar side of P's 5th metacarpal, tip at the hamate of the carpus. T's left hand grips radial side of P's hand, with fingers stabilizing the 4th metacarpal bone at the dorsal side. T's left thumb may support P's triquetral and hamate bones from the distal/palmar aspect.

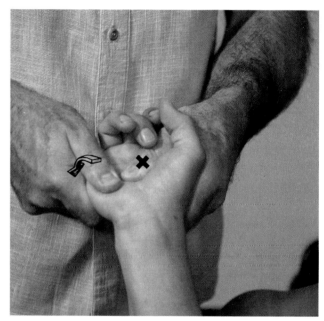

Fig. 64 a. Starting Position.

Procedure: Using this grip, T applies traction and gradually and fully *reposes* (extends and abducts) at the CMC joint of P's little finger.

Stimulation of Antagonists: T retains grip. T then asks P to move further in the direction of stretching, and resists that movement to stimulate P's antagonists.

Note: The opponens digiti minimi may be *maximally* stretched with P's elbow extended, forearm fully supinated, and wrist fully dorsally and radially flexed. However, this technique is more difficult to perform.

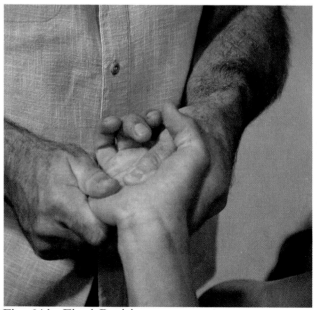

Fig. 64 b. Final Position.

PART 3

THERAPY TECHNIQUES FOR THE LOWER EXTREMITY

6 THE HIP

6.1 THERAPY GUIDE

The muscles which may restrict movement at the hip are listed in Table 6-1, along with the applicable therapies, indexed by manual section number and page. For the compound movements, some muscles listed may restrict only one or two components of the movement, but are listed as they act in the movement. Muscle actions are listed in Table 6-2.

In all cases, restriction at the hip may be regarded as affecting leg motion relative to the body, or conversely, body motion in the opposite direction relative to a stable leg. The various restrictions possible are listed in Movement Restriction Table 10.8 (p.172).

TABLE 6.1 Restrictions at the hip

SECTION	MOVEMENT RESTRICTED	RESTRICTING MUSCLE(S)	THERAPY	Number	Page
6.2	*Flexion with knee extended*	The Hamstrings: Biceps femoris, Semimembranosus, Semitendinosus		6.2.1	94
6.3	*Flexion with knee flexed*	Adductor magnus, Gluteus maximus and other adductors of hip		6.3.1	95
6.4	*Flexion, adduction and medial rotation*	Gluteus maximus		6.4.1, 6.5.1	96, 98
		The Hamstrings		6.2.1	94
		Piriformis		6.4.2	97
		Quadratus femoris		6.4.1	96
		Gluteus medius and minimus		6.10.1	107
6.5	*Flexion, adduction and lateral rotation*	Gluteus maximus, The Hamstrings, The Adductors		6.5.1	98
	other therapies for:	Gluteus maximus		6.4.1	96
		The Hamstrings		6.2.1	94
		Adductors		6.8.3, 6.11.1, 6.12.1-6.12.10	105,109, 110-119
6.6	*Flexion, abduction and medial rotation*	Gluteus maximus, The Hamstrings, The Adductors		6.6.1	99
	other therapies for:	Gluteus maximus		6.4.1	96
		The Hamstrings		6.2.1	94
		Adductors		6.8.3, 6.11.1, 6.12.1-6.12.10	105,109, 110-119
6.7	*Flexion, abduction and lateral rotation*	Gluteus medius, The Hamstrings, the Adductors		6.7.1	100
	other therapies for:	Gluteus medius		6.10.1	107
		The Hamstrings		6.2.1	94
		Adductors		6.8.3, 6.11.1, 6.12.1-6.12.10	105,109, 110-119
6.8	*Extension or hyperextension*	Iliopsoas		6.8.1, 6.11.1	101-102, 109
		Rectus femoris		6.8.2	103-104
		Pectineus		6.8.3	105
		Adductor longus and brevis		6.8.3, 6.11.1	105, 109
		Adductor magnus		6.8.3	105

6.9	*Extension/hyper-extension, adduction and medial rotation*	Gluteus medius and minimus	**6.10.1**	107
		Tensor fasciae latae	**6.10.2**	108
		Iliopsoas	**6.8.1, 6.11.1**	101-102, 109
		Sartorius	**6.9.1**	106
		Deep muscles of hip	**6.9.1**	106
6.10	*Extension/hyper-extension, adduction and lateral rotation*	Gluteus medius and minimus	**6.10.1**	107
		Tensor fasciae latae	**6.10.2**	108
6.11	*Extension/hyper-extension, abduction and medial rotation*	Pectineus	**6.8.3**	105
		Adductor brevis and longus	**6.11.1**	109
		Iliopsoas	**6.11.1, 6.8.1**	109, 101-102
6.12	*Extension/hyper-extension, abduction and lateral rotation*	Pectineus, Adductor magnus Gracilis, and Adductor brevis	**6.12.1-6.12.10**	110-119
	other therapies for:	Pectineus	**6.8.3**	105
		Adductor magnus	**6.8.3**	105
		Adductor brevis	**6.11.1**	109
6.13	*Medial rotation*	All lateral rotators	**6.13.1**	120-122
6.14	*Lateral rotation*	All medial rotators	**6.14.1**	123-125

NOTE: 1.   Other muscles listed in Table 10.8 (p.172) may also restrict.

TABLE 6.2 Actions of muscles which may restrict movements at the hip.

MUSCLE	ACTION
Muscles of the buttocks	
Gluteus maximus	Extends and laterally rotates at hip. Upper part: Abducts at hip. Lower part: Adducts at hip.
Gluteus medius	Ventral part: Flexes, abducts and medially rotates at hip. Middle part: abducts at hip Dorsal part: Extends, abducts and laterally rotates at hip.
Gluteus minimus	Ventral part: Flexes, abducts and medially rotates at hip. Middle part: Abducts at hip Dorsal part: Extends, abducts and laterally rotates at hip.
Tensor fasciae latae	Abducts, flexes and medially rotates at hip. Extends and laterally rotates at knee.
Piriformis	Abducts, laterally rotates and extends at hip (to about 60o flexion).
Quadratus femoris	Laterally rotates, extends and adducts at hip.
Muscles of the thigh The "Hamstrings"	
Biceps femoris	Long head: Flexes and laterally rotates at knee. Extends, laterally rotates and adducts at hip. Short head: Flexes and laterally rotates at knee.
Semimembranosus	Flexes and medially rotates at knee. Extends, adducts and medially rotates at hip.
Semitendinosus	Flexes and medially rotates at knee. Extends, adducts and medially rotates at hip.
Adductor brevis	Adducts, laterally rotates and flexes at hip.
Adductor longus	Adducts, laterally rotates and flexes at hip.
Adductor magnus	Extends and adducts at hip. Part with origin at ischial tuberosity: Adducts, extends and medially rotates at hip.
Iliopsoas	Ventral and lateral flexes lumbar spine. Flexes and laterally rotates at hip; abducts or adducts (depending on which extreme position hip is in).
Rectus femoris	Flexes at hip. Extends at knee.
Pectineus	Flexes, adducts and laterally rotates at hip.
Sartorius	Flexes, abducts and laterally rotates at hip. Flexes and medially rotates at knee.
Gracilis	Adducts at hip. Flexes and laterally rotates when hip is extended. Extends and medially rotates when hip is maximally flexed. Flexes and medially rotates at knee.

6.2.1. Therapy for the **biceps femoris**, **semimembranosus** and **semitendinosus** (The **Hamstrings**).

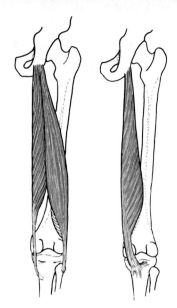

Starting Position: P: Supine; hip in full flexion and thigh stabilized with a belt; knee extended as much as shortened muscles allow. T: Standing at P's right side, facing P's head.

Grip: P's heel and lower leg rest on T's left shoulder. T's left hand grips ventral side of P's lower leg just below the knee. T's right hand stabilizes P's left thigh ventrally just proximal to the knee, or left thigh may be stabilized with a belt.

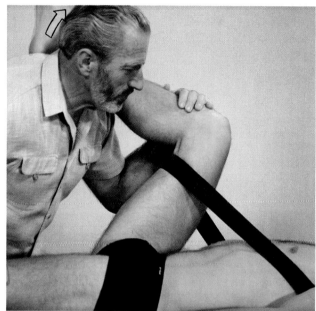

Procedure: Using this grip, T gradually and fully *extends* at P's knee.

Fig. 65 a. Starting Position.

Stimulation of Antagonists: T moves left hand just proximal to P's right ankle. T then asks P to move further in the direction of stretching, and resists that movement to stimulate P's antagonists.

Notes: This technique is easier for T and more comfortable for P than conventional stretching with extended knee. It may be used in all cases where hip flexion is greater with the knee flexed than with the knee extended.

For *maximal* stretching of the **Hamstrings**:

Muscle	Technique
Biceps femoris	Same, except P's leg is *medially rotated* at both hip and knee and *adducted* at hip.
Semimembranosus and semitendinosus	Same, except P's leg is *laterally rotated* at both hip and knee and *abducted* at hip.

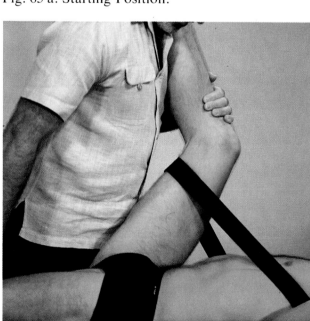

Fig. 65 b. Final Position.

6.3.1. Therapy for the **extensor muscles**, *except* the **Hamstrings**.

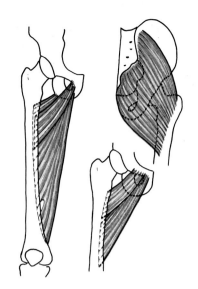

Starting Position: P: Supine; left leg stabilized with a belt across his thigh just above the knee; right hip and knee in flexion. T: Standing at P's right side, facing P's head.

Grip: T's left hand grips ventral side of P's knee. T's right hand grips P's thigh from the dorsal/medial side just above the knee. (This will also protect the knee when maximal flexion is painful).

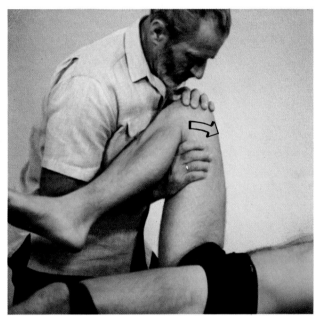

Fig. 66 a. Starting Position.

Procedure: Using this grip, T gradually and fully *flexes* at P's hip.

Stimulation of Antagonists: T reverses grip. T then asks P to move further in the direction of stretching, and resists that movement with left hand to stimulate P's antagonists.

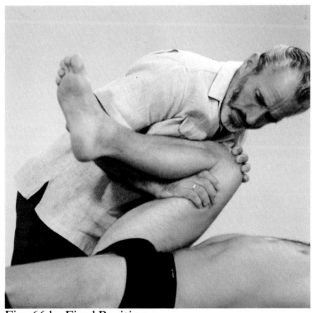

Fig. 66 b. Final Position.

6.4.1. Therapy for the **extensors, abductors** and **lateral rotators.**

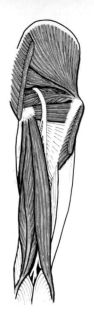

Starting Position: P: Supine; left leg extended with left thigh stabilized by a belt; right hip and knee in flexion. T: Standing at P's right side, facing P's head.

Grip: T's left hand grips ventral side of P's knee. T's right hand grips medial side of P's heel or lower leg just above the ankle.

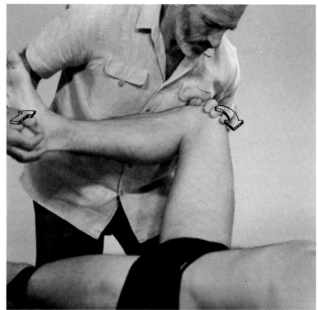

Fig. 67 a. Starting Position.

Procedure: Using this grip, T gradually and fully *flexes, adducts* and *medially rotates* at P's hip.

Stimulation of Antagonists: T retains grip. T then asks P to move further in the direction of stretching, and resists that movement to stimulate P's antagonists.

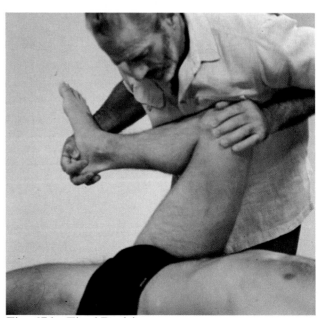

Fig. 67 b. Final Position.

96

6.4.2. Therapy for the **extensors, abductors** and **lateral rotators.** *Hip flexed 60°.* (Mainly stretching the **piriformis**).

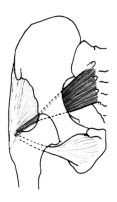

Starting Position: P: Supine; pelvis stabilized with a belt; left hip and knee extended; right hip and knee positioned in approximately 60° flexion; right foot steadied against the couch on the lateral side of left leg. T: Standing at P's right side, facing P's head.

Grip: T's right hand grips ventral-lateral side of P's knee. T's left hand and forearm support and control P's pelvis.

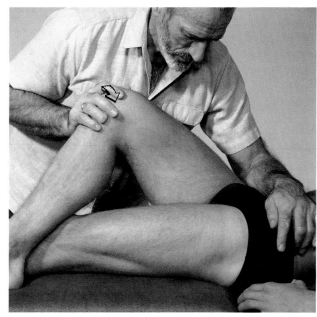

Fig. 68 a. Starting Position.

Procedure: Using this grip, T gradually and fully *adducts* at P's hip.

Stimulation of Antagonists: T retains grip. T then asks P to move further in the direction of stretching, and resists that movement to stimulate P's antagonists.

Note: P's left thigh may limit movement of the right leg. So to attain maximal stretching of the **piriformis,** it may be necessary to flex P's left knee and flex and abduct the left hip before to further adducting the right hip.

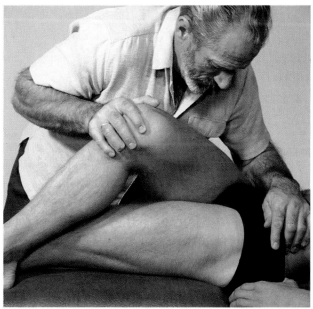

Fig. 68 b. Final Position.

6.5.1. Therapy for the **extensors, abductors and medial rotators.**

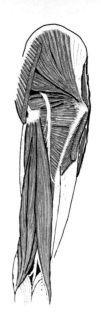

Starting Position: P: Supine; left thigh and pelvis stabilized with belts; right hip and knee flexed. T: Standing at P's right side, level with P's hips.

Grip: T's left hand grips ventral side of P's knee. T's right hand grips P's lower leg just above the ankle.

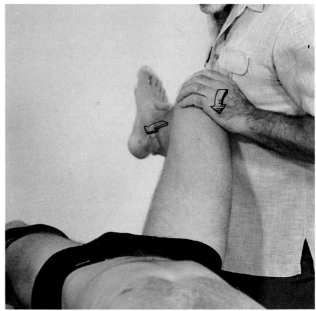

Fig. 69 a. Starting Position.

Procedure: Using this grip, T gradually and fully *flexes*, *adducts* and *laterally rotates* at P's hip.

Stimulation of Antagonists: T retains grip. T then asks P to move further in the direction of stretching, and resists that movement to stimulate P's antagonists.

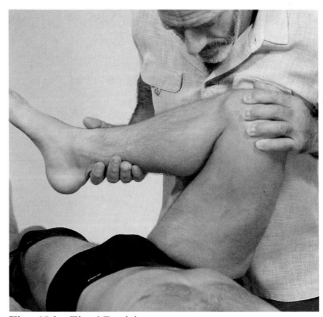

Fig. 69 b. Final Position.

6.6.1. Therapy for the **extensors, adductors and lateral rotators.**

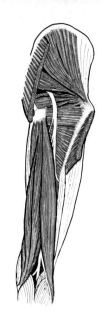

Starting Position: P: Supine; left thigh stabilized with a belt; (a belt over P's pelvis provides additional stabilization); right hip and knee flexed. T: Standing at P's right side, level with P's knee.

Grip: T's left hand grips medial side of P's thigh just above the knee. T's right hand grips P's lower leg just above the ankle.

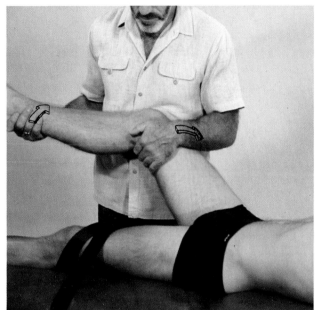

Fig. 70 a. Starting Position.

Procedure: Using this grip, T gradually and fully *flexes*, *abducts* and *medially rotates* at P's hip.

Stimulation of Antagonists: T moves right hand to proximal-lateral side of knee. T then asks P to move further in the direction of stretching, and resists that movement with both hands to stimulate P's antagonists.

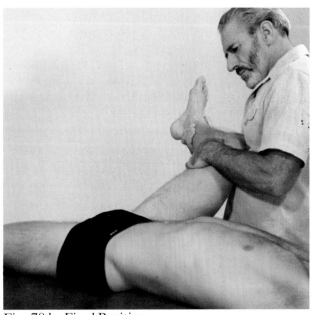

Fig. 70 b. Final Position.

6.7.1. Therapy for the **extensors, adductors and medial rotators.**

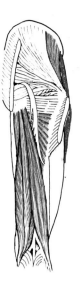

Starting Position: P: Supine; left thigh stabilized with a belt; (a belt over P's pelvis provides additional stabilization); right hip and knee flexed. T: Standing at P's right side, facing P's head.

Grip: T's left hand grips ventral side of P's knee. T's right hand grips P's lower leg just above the ankle.

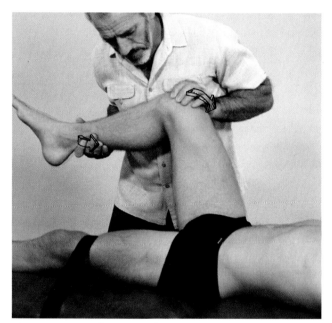

Fig. 71 a. Starting Position.

Procedure: Using this grip, T gradually and fully *flexes, abducts* and *laterally rotates* at P's hip.

Stimulation of Antagonists: T retains grip. T then asks P to move further in the direction of stretching, and resists that movement to stimulate P's antagonists.

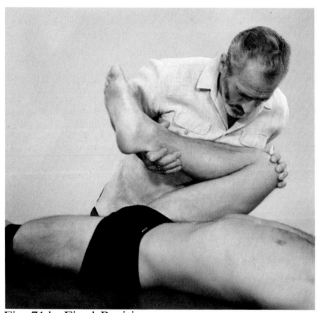

Fig. 71 b. Final Position.

6.8.1A. Therapy for the **iliopsoas.** *Muscle markedly shortened.*

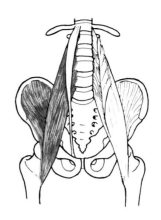

Starting Position: P: Prone with hip joint located sightly forward of couch hinge (so lower end of couch may be elevated); left leg over side of couch, foot on the floor; to avoid lumbar lordosis (which also may be painful), the foot may be moved forward on the floor and stabilized in position by T's left foot. This flexes hip further, flattens the lordosis and prevents P evading the stretching; a cushion may be placed under the abdomen to increase ventral flexion of the lumbar spine (and therefore the effect of the stretching); pelvis stabilized with a belt. T: Standing facing P's left side about level with P's right knee.

Grip: T's right hand adjusts the angle of the foot end of the couch. T's left hand is placed on the dorsal side of P's right thigh just distal to the ischial tuberosity.

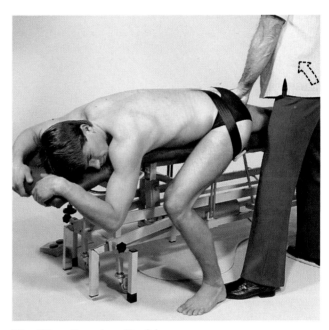

Fig. 72 a. Starting Position.

Procedure: Using this grip, T's right hand slowly lifts the lower part of the couch, thereby gradually and fully *extending* at P's hip.

Stimulation of Antagonists: T moves right hand to dorsal side of thigh just proximal to knee. T then asks P to move further in the direction of stretching, and resists that movement to stimulate P's antagonists. To increase contraction when stimulating, T uses left hand to slap P's right buttock.

Note: If the lower end of the couch cannot be elevated, T can use right hand to support P's leg just above the knee, and gradually lift the leg to extend at the hip.

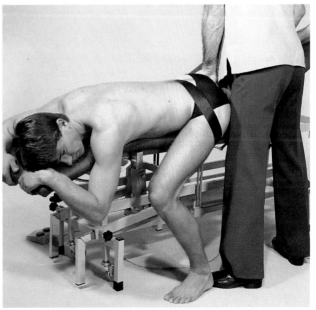

Fig. 72 b. Final Position.

6.8.1B. Therapy for the **iliopsoas.** *Maximal stretching.*

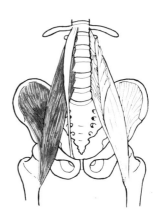

Starting Position: P: Prone; trunk in left lateral flexion; left leg over side of couch with foot on floor; to avoid lumbar lordosis (which may be painful), foot may be moved forward on the floor and stabilized in position by T's left foot; this flexes hip further, flattens the lordosis and prevents P evading the stretching; left foot position regulates lumbar lordosis, important in treating patients with low back pain; a cushion may be placed under the abdomen to increase ventral flexion of the lumbar spine (and therefore the effect of the stretching); pelvis stabilized with a belt; right knee flexed with right hip in full medial rotation. T: Standing oblique, facing P's left side level with P's thighs.

Grip: T's right hand grips P's lower leg just above the ankle. After raising lower end of couch (see Procedure), T's left hand can be used to stabilize P's right thigh at the dorsal side just distal to the ischial tuberosity; this increases stretching.

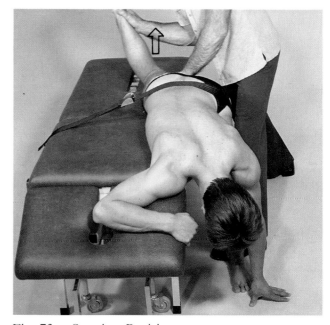

Fig. 73 a. Starting Position.

Procedure: Using this grip, T uses left hand to slowly raise the foot end of the couch, thereby gradually and fully *extending medially rotated* hip.

Stimulation of Antagonists: T moves right hand to dorsal side of thigh just proximal to knee. T then asks P to move further in the direction of stretching, and resists that movement to stimulate P's antagonists. To increase contraction when stimulating, T uses left hand to slap P's right buttock.

Note: If the belt stabilization fails to hold P's pelvis in place after the foot end of the couch is raised, T's left hand can be placed over P's right thigh to press the pelvis ventrally towards the couch.

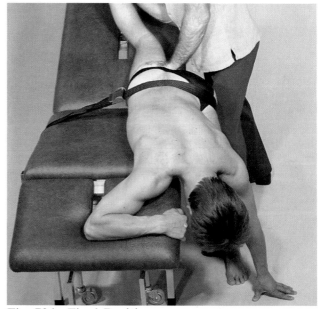

Fig. 73 b. Final Position.

6.8.2A Therapy for the **rectus femoris.**
Muscle markedly shortened.

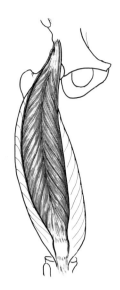

Starting Position: P: Prone; pelvis (and thus the origin of the rectus femoris) stabilized to the couch with a belt; left leg over side of couch with foot on floor; to avoid lumbar lordosis (which also may be painful), foot can be moved forward on floor and stabilized in position by T's left foot; this flexes P's hip further, flattens the lordosis and prevents P from evading the stretching; a cushion may be placed under P's abdomen to increase ventral flexion of the lumbar spine (and therefore the effect of the stretching); right knee flexed. T: Standing facing P's left side at the lower end of the couch.

Grip: T's right hand grips ventral side of P's ankle. T's left hand stabilizes P's thigh just distal to the ischial tuberosity.

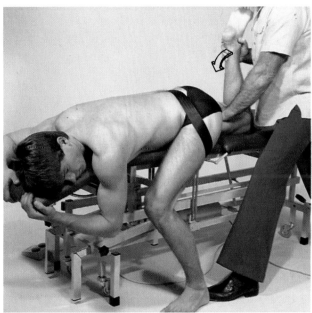

Fig. 74 a. Starting Position.

Procedure: Using this grip, T gradually and fully *flexes* at P's knee until the heel reaches the buttock.

Note: Stimulation of the antagonists: *Not recommended; may cause cramps.*

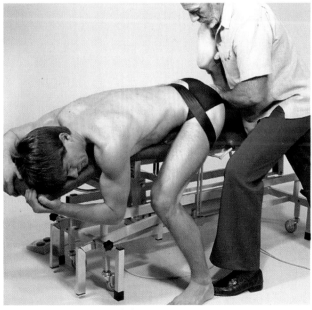

Fig. 74 b. Final Position.

6.8.2B. Therapy for the **rectus femoris.** *Maximal stretching.*

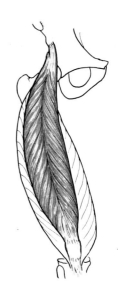

Starting Position: P: Prone; pelvis (and thus the origin of the rectus femoris) stabilized to the couch with a belt; left leg over side of couch with foot on floor; to avoid lumbar lordosis (which also may be painful), foot can be moved forward on floor and stabilized in position by T's left foot; this flexes P's hip further, flattens the lordosis and prevents P from evading the stretching; a cushion may be placed under P's abdomen to increase ventral flexion of the lumbar spine (and therefore the effect of the stretching); right hip held in full hyperextension by raising the foot end of the couch; right knee flexed. T: Standing oblique, facing P's left side at the lower end of the couch.

Grip: T's right hand grips ventral side of P's ankle. T's left hand stabilizes P's thigh just distal to the ischial tuberosity.

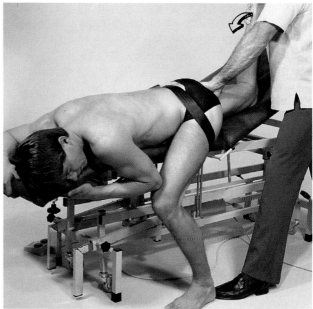

Fig. 75 a. Starting Position.

Procedure: Using this grip, T gradually and fully *flexes* at P's knee until the heel reaches the buttock.

Notes: Stimulation of the antagonists: *Not recommended; may cause cramps.*

Once in the final position, further stretching may be attained by gradually raising the foot end of the couch higher.

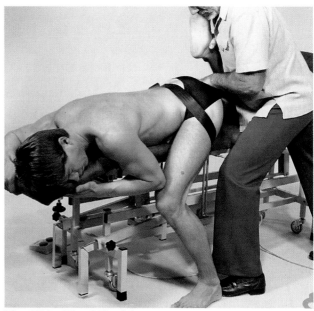

Fig. 75 b. Final Position.

6.8.3. Therapy for the **pectineus** and **adductor longus, brevis and magnus.**

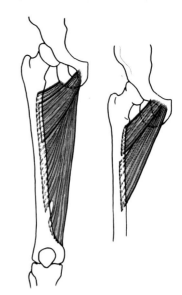

Starting Position: P: Lying on left side; left hip and knee fully flexed (or P holding own left knee with both hands), pelvis stabilized with a belt just cranial to the greater trochanter; right hip fully extended and medially rotated. T: Standing behind P, level with P's thigh.

Grip: T's right hand grips the medial side of P's knee and T's arm supports P's lower leg. T's left hand placed on P's pelvis at belt, just cranial to the greater trochanter, to stabilize and control P's pelvis.

Procedure: Using this grip, T gradually and fully *abducts* at P's hip.

Stimulation of Antagonists: T moves left hand to lateral side of thigh proximal to the knee, and right hand to lateral side of leg just proximal to the ankle. T then asks P to move further in the direction of stretching, and resists that movement to stimulate P's antagonists.

Notes: Abduction at the hip may be performed in varying degrees of flexion, extension and lateral or medial rotation as needed. However, accordingly it may be necessary to change both the starting position and the grip.

Maximal extension, abduction, and medial rotation at the hip (when none of the surrounding tissues are shortened) produces a *close packed position* which blocks further movement.

With the knee extended, the short **adductors** and the **gracilis** are stretched if the hip is also fully extended, abducted and laterally rotated. Flexing the knee excludes the **gracilis** from stretching.

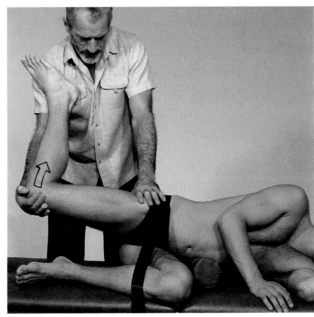

Fig. 76 a. Starting Position.

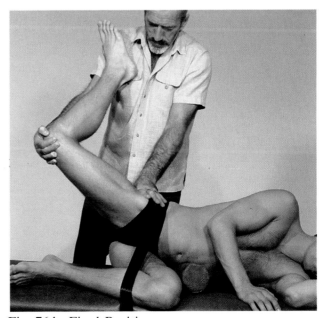

Fig. 76 b. Final Position.

6.9.1.   Therapy for the **deep muscles**.

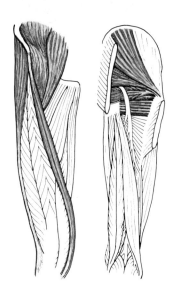

Starting Position: P: Lying on right side; left hip and knee both flexed approximately 90° with knee, lower leg and foot resting on couch or on cushion; right hip fully extended with knee flexed approximately 90°; pelvis stabilized with a belt; cushion may be placed under waist to further support pelvis and lumbar spine. T: Standing behind P at the lower end of the couch, about level with P's thigh.

Grip: T's right hand grips P's right knee and thigh from the ventral/lateral side. T's left hand grips P's lower leg just above the ankle.

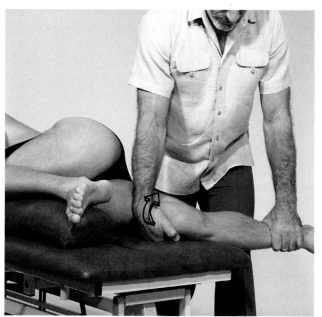

Fig. 77 a. Starting Position.

Procedure: Using this grip, T gradually and fully *extends*, *adducts* and *medially rotates* at P's hip.

Stimulation of Antagonists: T retains grip. T then asks P to move further in the direction of stretching, and resists that movement to stimulate P's antagonists.

Notes: The **iliopsoas, gluteus medius and minimus** and **tensor fasciae latae** are also stretched slightly in procedure, see therapies 6.8.1A, B pp. 101-102.

The **sartorius** may be stretched using this technique, if P's right knee is extended instead of flexed.

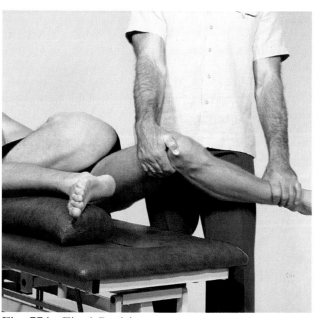

Fig. 77 b. Final Position.

6.10.1. Therapy for the **gluteus medius and minimus.**

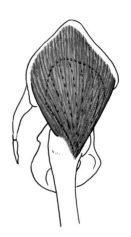

Starting Position: P: Lying on right side; left hip and knee flexed approximately 90° with knee, lower leg and foot resting on couch or a pillow; right hip and knee extended; pelvis stabilized with a belt; if necessary, a firm cushion may be placed under the waist to further support the pelvis and lumbar spine. T: Standing behind P at the lower end of the couch, level with P's right knee.

Grip: T's left hand grips P's ankle and the proximal part of the foot at the dorsal-lateral side (or around P's lower leg just above the ankle). T's right hand grips ventral-lateral side of P's thigh just above the knee.

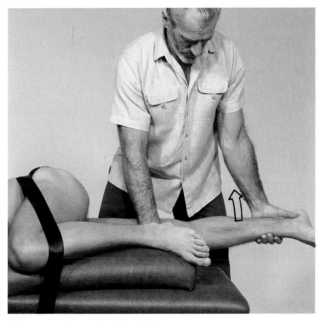

Fig. 78 a. Starting Position.

Procedure: Using this grip, T gradually and fully *adducts* at P's hip.

Stimulation of Antagonists: T moves hands to medial side of P's thigh and leg. T then asks P to move further in the direction of stretching, and resists that movement to stimulate P's antagonists.

Notes: To completely stretch the **gluteus medius and minimus,** the above procedure should be repeated with the following modifications:

Specific stretching of parts of the **gluteus medius and minimus:**

Ventral part	Same grip and procedure, except P's hip is also *extended* and *laterally rotated.*
Dorsal part	Same grip and procedure, except P's hip is also slightly *flexed* and *medially rotated.*

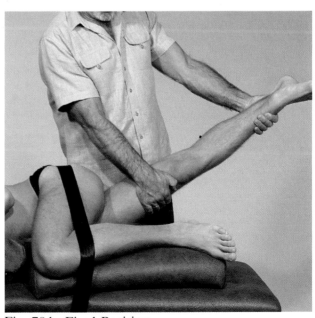

Fig. 78 b. Final Position.

6.10.2.   Therapy for the **tensor fasciae latae.**

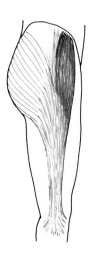

Starting Position: P: Lying on right side; left hip and knee flexed approximately 90° with knee, lower leg and foot resting on couch or pillow; right hip extended and laterally rotated with knee flexed approximately 90°; pelvis stabilized with a belt; firm cushion under waist improves support of pelvis and lumbar spine. T: Standing behind P, level with P's upper leg.

Grip: T's left hand grips ventral-lateral side of P's knee and thigh and forearm supports lateral side of P's lower leg. T's right hand stabilizes and controls P's pelvis.

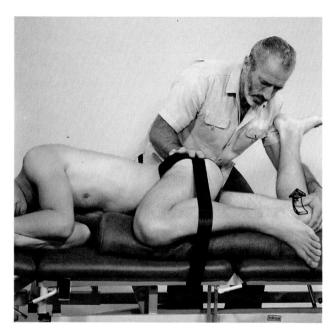

Fig. 79 a. Starting Position.

Procedure: Using this grip, T gradually and fully *extends*, *adducts* and *laterally rotates* at P's hip.

Stimulation of Antagonists: T moves right hand to medial-dorsal side of thigh just proximal to the knee. T then asks P to move further in the direction of stretching, and resists that movement to stimulate P's antagonists.

Note: Maximal stretching is attained when P's right knee is flexed maximally.

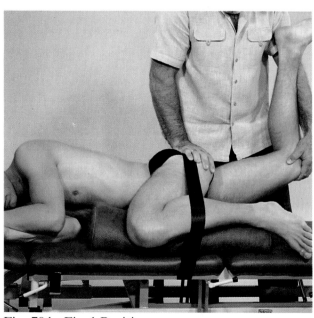

Fig. 79 b. Final Position.

6.11.1. Therapy for the **pectineus, adductor brevis, adductor longus** and **iliopsoas.**

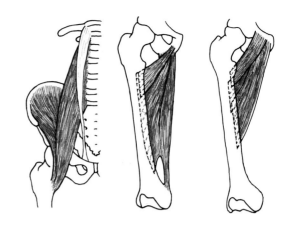

Starting Position: P: Prone; if necessary, a cushion may be placed under abdomen to stabilize pelvis and lumbar spine; pelvis is then stabilized with a belt. T: Standing facing P's right side.

Grip: T's left hand holds ventral-medial side of P's knee and thigh, and P's lower leg is stabilized between T's left arm and chest. T's right hand stabilizes P's right ilium.

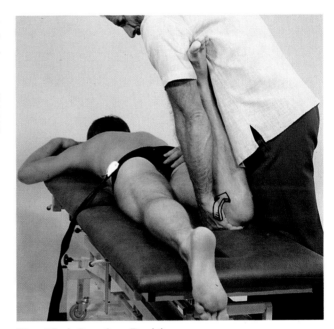

Fig. 80 a. Starting Position.

Procedure: Using this grip, T gradually and fully *extends, medially rotates* and *abducts* at P's hip.

Stimulation of Antagonists: T moves right hand to dorsal side of P's thigh just proximal to knee and left hand to lateral side of leg just proximal to the ankle. T then asks P to move further in the direction of stretching, and resists that movement to stimulate P's antagonists.

Notes: For more secure pelvis stabilization, T positions P's left leg over the edge of the couch with the sole of the foot on the floor. This also flexes P's lumbar spine.

To increase the stretching, the lower part of the couch may be raised. However, T must then alter grip, see therapy 6.8.1A, p. 101.

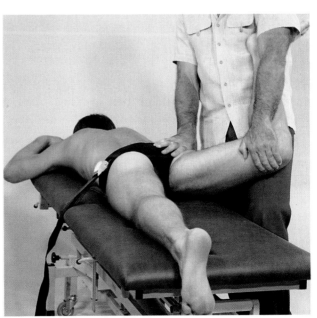

Fig. 80 b. Final Position.

6.12.1.   Therapy for the **adductor muscles.**
Bilateral stretching.

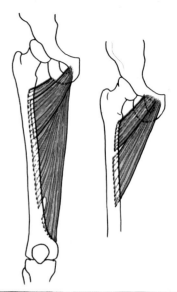

Starting Position: P: Supine; hips and knees flexed with feet together on couch; to prevent lordosis, lumbar spine should be flexed either by placing a cushion under the thorax or by raising the head end of the couch; pelvis stabilized with a belt. T: Standing oblique, at the lower end of the couch, level with P's feet.

Grip: Using both hands, T grips ventral-medial sides of P's knees. For extra force, T's forearm(s) may be placed against P's knee(s), as shown here for right hand and forearm.

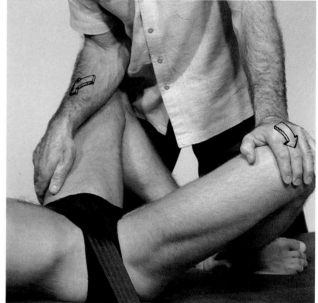

Fig. 81 a. Starting Position.

Procedure: Using this grip, T gradually and fully *abducts* at P's hips.

Stimulation of Antagonists: T moves hands to lateral sides of knees. T then asks P to move further in the direction of stretching, and resists that movement to stimulate P's antagonists.

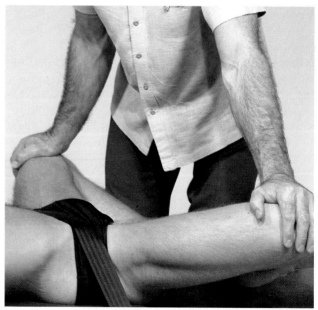

Fig. 81 b. Final Position.

6.12.2. Therapy for the **adductors.** *Hip extended.*

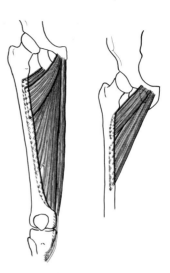

Starting Position: P: Supine; right leg extended; left hip extended and abducted; pelvis stabilized with a belt; left lower leg over side of couch further stabilizes pelvis; to prevent lordosis, lumbar spine should be flexed either by a cushion under thorax or by raising the head end of the couch. T: Standing at lower end of couch, facing P's right side.

Grip: T's right hand grips P's lower leg just above the ankle. T's left hand grips medial-dorsal side of P's thigh just above the knee.

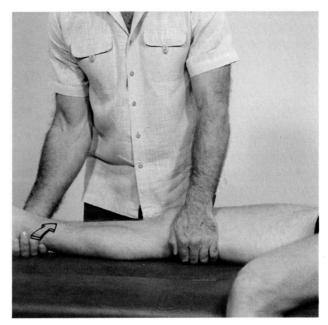

Fig. 82 a. Starting Position.

Procedure: Using this grip, T gradually and fully *abducts* at P's hip.

Stimulation of Antagonists: T moves left hand to lateral side of P's thigh proximal to the knee. T then asks P to move further in the direction of stretching, and resists that movement to stimulate P's antagonists.

Note: For *maximal* stretching, T can medially or laterally rotate (as needed) while abducting at P's hip. P's hip must not be flexed during abduction.

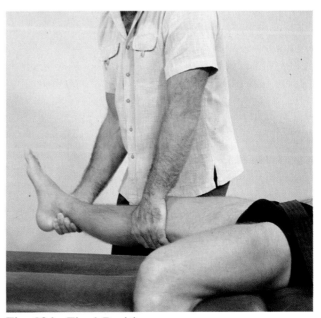

Fig. 82 b. Final Position.

111

6.12.3.   Therapy for the **adductors**. (Mainly stretching the **long adductors**, *except the gracilis*). *Hip flexed 45°.*

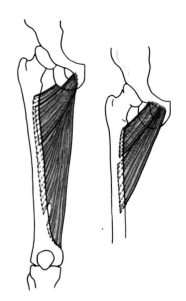

Starting Position: P: Supine; right hip flexed approximately 45° with foot on couch; left hip extended and abducted; belt stabilizing pelvis; left lower leg over side of couch further stabilizes pelvis; to prevent lordosis, lumbar spine should be flexed either by a cushion under the thorax or by raising the head end of the couch. T: Standing facing P's right side.

Grip: T's right hand grips medial side of P's lower leg just above the ankle; right forearm lying along the medial side of P's lower leg and knee. T's left hand stabilizes and controls P's pelvis on the opposite side.

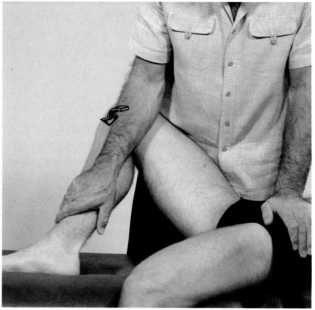

Fig. 83 a. Starting Position.

Procedure: Using this grip, T gradually and fully *abducts* at P's hip.

Stimulation of Antagonists: T moves right hand to lateral side of P's right knee. T then asks P to move further in the direction of stretching, and resists that movement to stimulate P's antagonists.

Note: T can vary abduction, as needed, by varying position of P's foot on couch.

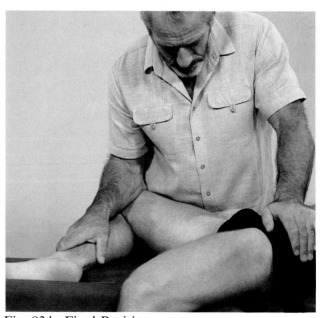

Fig. 83 b. Final Position.

6.12.4. Therapy for the **adductors.** *Hip flexed 90°.*

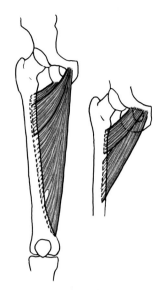

Starting Position: P: Supine; right knee flexed; right hip flexed approximately 90°; left hip extended and abducted; belt stabilizing pelvis; left lower leg may be over side of couch to further stabilize pelvis; to prevent lordosis, lumbar spine should be flexed either by a cushion under the thorax or by raising the head end of couch. T: Standing at P's right side.

Grip: T's right hand grips P's foot or lower leg just above the ankle, right forearm lying along the medial side of P's lower leg and knee. T's left hand stabilizes and controls P's pelvis on the opposite side.

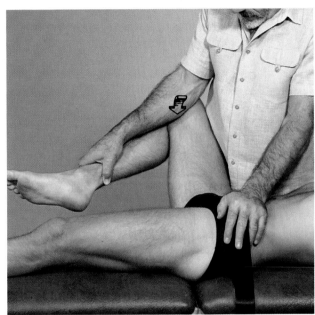

Fig. 84 a. Starting Position.

Procedure: Using this grip, T gradually and fully *abducts* at P's hip.

Stimulation of Antagonists: T moves right hand to lateral side of P's right knee. T then asks P to move further in the direction of stretching, and resists that movement to stimulate P's antagonists.

Notes: T should stretch with P's hip rotated to the position where abduction is most restricted.

From hyperextension to approximately 60° flexion, the adductors act as *flexors* and laterally rotators at the hip and are maximally stretched when the hip is extended, abducted and *medially* rotated.

From 60° flexion to full flexion, the adductors act as *extensors* and medial rotators at the hip and are maximally stretched when the hip is flexed, abducted and *laterally* rotated.

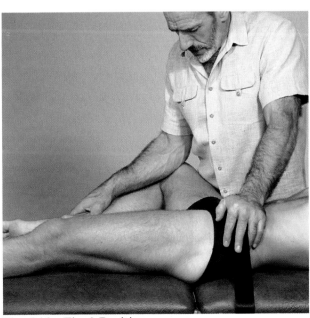

Fig. 84 b. Final Position.

6.12.5.   Therapy for the **adductors.** *Hip fully flexed.*

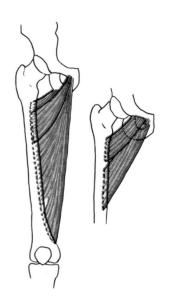

Starting Position: P: Supine; right hip fully flexed; left hip extended and abducted; belt stabilizing pelvis; left lower leg may be positioned over side of couch to further stabilize pelvis; to prevent lordosis, lumbar spine should be flexed either by a cushion under the thorax or by raising the head end of the couch. T: Standing, left side towards P's right side.

Grip: T's right hand grips P's lower leg just above the ankle, right forearm lying along the medial side of P's lower leg and knee. T's left hand stabilizes and controls P's pelvis on the opposite side.

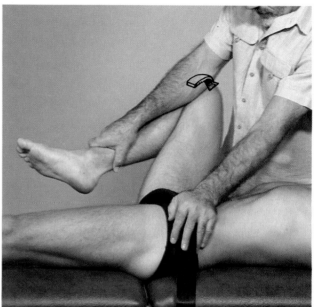

Fig. 85 a. Starting Position.

Procedure: Using this grip, T gradually and fully *abducts* at P's hip.

Stimulation of Antagonists: T moves right hand to lateral side of P's right knee. T then asks P to move further in the direction of stretching, and resists that movement to stimulate P's antagonists.

Note: For increased stretching effect while abducting, T may laterally rotate P's hip, to the degree needed and possible.

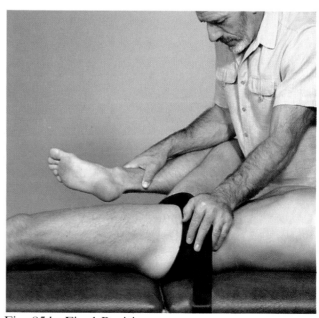

Fig. 85 b. Final Position.

6.12.6. Therapy for the **adductors. (Mainly stretching the long adductors,** *except the gracilis). Hip flexed 45°.*

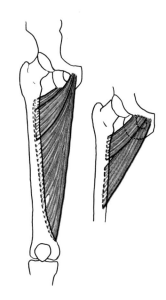

Starting Position: P: Prone; hip flexed approximately 45°; knee flexed approximately 90°. T: Standing facing P's left side.

Grip: T's right hand controls degree of rotation at P's hip by gripping P's lower leg just above the ankle and stabilizing it against P's left leg. T's left hand is placed over P's right greater trochanter.

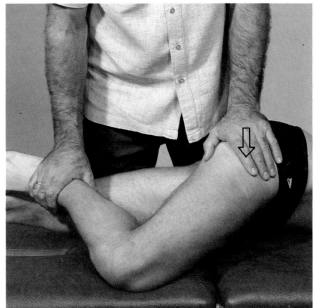

Fig. 86 a. Starting Position.

Procedure: Using this grip, T pushes left hand down to gradually and fully *abduct* at P's hip; P's pelvis rotates until the medial side of the thigh is pressed against the couch.

Stimulation of Antagonists: T moves right hand to lateral side of P's knee and left hand to ventral side of thigh just distal to hip. T then asks P to move further in the direction of stretching, and resists that movement to stimulate P's antagonists.

Note: If needed, T may tension a belt at the level of P's greater trochanter to draw the thigh down to the couch, see therapy 6.12.9 p. 118.

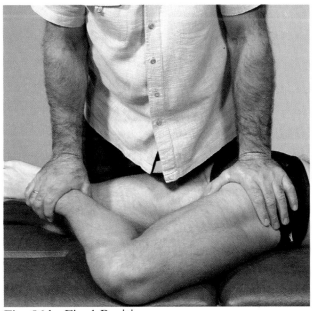

Fig. 86 b. Final Position.

115

6.12.7. Therapy for the **adductors**. *Hip flexed 90°.*

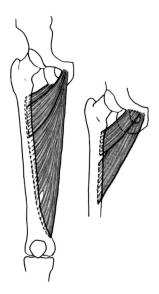

Starting Position: P: Prone; hip and knee flexed approximately 90°. T: Standing facing P's left side.

Grip: T's right hand controls degree of rotation at P's hip by gripping P's lower leg just proximal to the ankle and stabilizing it against the couch. T's left hand is placed over P's right greater trochanter.

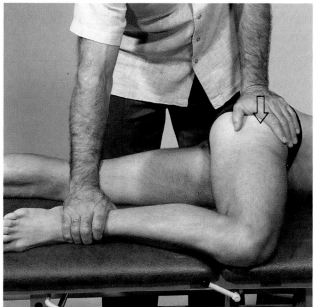

Fig. 87 a. Starting Position.

Procedure: Using this grip, T pushes left hand down to gradually and fully abduct at P's hip. P's pelvis rotates until the medial side of the thigh is pressed against the couch.

Stimulation of Antagonists: T moves right hand to lateral side of P's right knee and left hand to ventral side of thigh just distal to hip. T then asks P to move further in the direction of stretching, and resists that movement to stimulate P's antagonists.

Note: If needed, T may tension a belt at the level of P's greater trochanter to draw the thigh down to the couch, see therapy 6.12.9 p. 118.

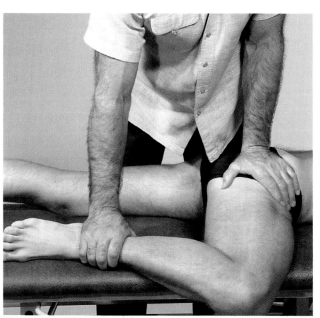

Fig. 87 b. Final Position.

6.12.8.   Therapy for the **adductors**. *Hip fully flexed.*

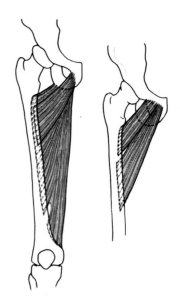

Starting Position: P: Prone; hip fully flexed; knee flexed approximately 130°. T: Standing facing P's left side.

Grip: T's right hand controls degree of rotation at P's hip by gripping P's lower leg just above the ankle and stabilizing it against the couch. T's left hand is placed over P's right greater trochanter.

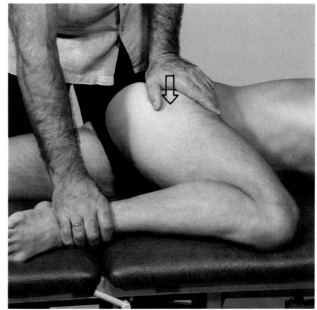

Fig. 88 a. Starting Position.

Procedure: Using this grip, T pushes left hand down to gradually and fully *abduct* at P's hip. P's pelvis rotates until the medial side of the thigh is pressed against the couch.

Stimulation of Antagonists: T moves right hand to lateral side of P's right knee and left hand to ventral side of thigh just distal to the hip. T then asks P to move further in the direction of stretching, and resists that movement to stimulate P's antagonists.

Note: If needed, T may tension a belt at the level of P's greater trochanter to draw the thigh down to the couch, see therapy 6.12.9 p. 118.

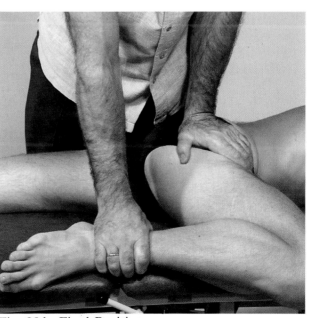

Fig. 88 b. Final Position.

6.12.9. Therapy for the **adductors.** *Belt tension alternative to preceding three therapies.*

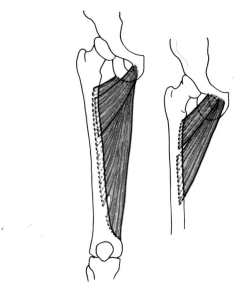

Alternative technique: If P is large and/or strong compared to T, or T otherwise finds pressing P's thigh down to the couch difficult, then belt tension may be used instead of T's to apply the force required for abduction in therapies 6.12.6, 6.12.7, and 6.12.8 on the preceding three pages. The example shown here is the alternate belt procedure to the hand procedure of therapy 6.12.6 on page 115.

Starting Position: P: As specified for the technique involved, except P's pelvis is stabilized to the couch with a belt having a continuously-adjustable buckle, with the free tongue of the belt lying over P's left side, towards T.

Grip: T's left hand grips the buckle of the belt. T's right hand holds the free tongue of the belt near the buckle.

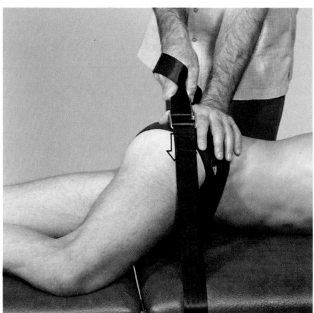

Fig. 89 a. Starting Position.

Procedure: T tightens the belt. T asks P to push upwards against the belt,.
This force adducts the right hip. T then asks P to relax slowly. As P relaxes, T further tightens the belt to gradually *abduct* at P's hip. P's pelvis then rotates so the medial side of the right thigh and hip are gradually pressed down against the couch. T repeats until maximal stretching is attained.

Stimulation of Antagonists: Same as for preceding three techniques: T moves right hand to lateral side of P's right knee and left hand to ventral side of thigh just distal to hip. T then asks P to move further in the direction of stretching, and resists that movement to stimulate P's antagonists.

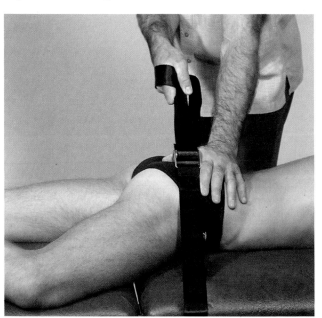

Fig. 89 b. Final Position.

6.12.10. Therapy for the **adductors** (including the **gracilis**). *P on side.*

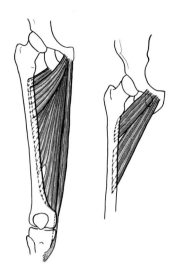

Starting Position: P: Lying on left side; left hip and knee fully flexed; right leg extended; pelvis stabilized by a belt; P may hold own left knee with both hands (this helps prevent lordosis). T: Standing behind P at the lower end of the couch.

Grip: T's right hand grips medial-dorsal side of P's ankle. T's left hand grips P's thigh from behind just above the knee and from the medial-ventral side.

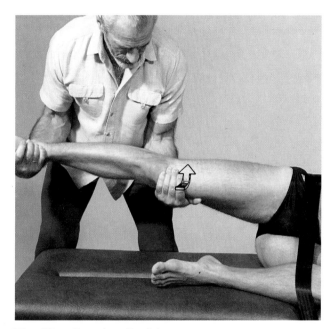

Fig. 90 a. Starting Position.

Procedure: Using this grip, T gradually and fully *abducts*, *medially rotates* and *extends* at P's hip.

Stimulation of Antagonists: T moves both hands to lateral sides of leg. T then asks P to move further in the direction of stretching, and resists that movement to stimulate P's antagonists.

Notes: Flexing the knee excludes the gracilis from stretching, as in therapy 6.8.3 p. 105. As the exact function of the adductors depends on hip position always stretch in position of maximum restriction.

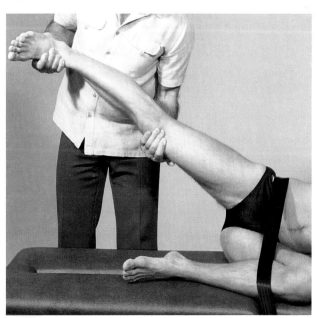

Fig. 90 b. Final Position.

119

6.13.1A. Therapy for the **lateral rotator muscles.** *Knee normal, flexed 90° in treatment.*

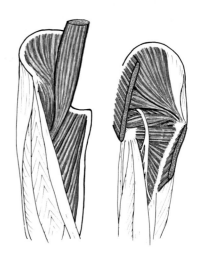

Starting Position: P: Prone; knee flexed 90°; pelvis stabilized with a belt. T: Standing facing P's right side.

Grip: T's left hand grips ventral-medial side of P's knee and thigh; left forearm lies along the medial side of P's lower leg. T's right hand stabilizes and controls P's right ilium and sacrum.

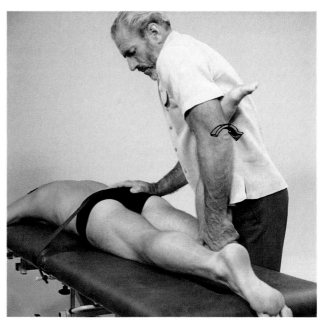

Procedure: Using this grip, T gradually and fully *medially rotates* at P's hip.

Fig. 91 a. Starting Position.

Stimulation of Antagonists: T may change grip or retain grip and use body to resist motion. T asks P to move further in the direction of stretching, and resists that movement to stimulate P's antagonists.

Notes: The above procedure assumes a normal knee capable of tolerating stress when flexed. In some cases, the knee may be so painful and/or unstable that stress should not be applied to a flexed knee, or, in the extreme, not be applied to the knee at all. T must then alter grip and procedure accordingly.
See the following two therapies, 6.13.1B and 6.13.1C, pages 121 and 122.

As medial rotation improves with treatment, the hip may successively be abducted more in the starting position.

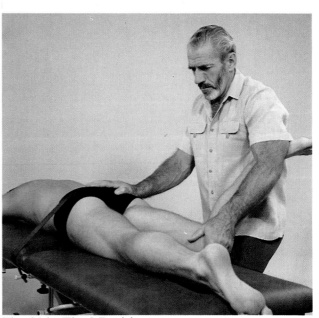

Fig. 91 b. Final Position.

6.13.1B Therapy for the **lateral rotator muscles.** *Alternative technique, for knees tolerating stress only if extended.*

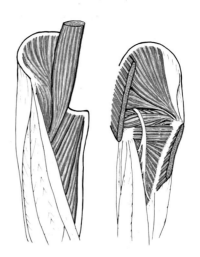

Starting Position: P: Prone; pelvis stabilized with a belt. T: Standing between P's legs at the foot of the couch, facing P's head.

Grip: T's left hand grips ventral side of P's thigh just above the knee, and T's right hand grips the dorsal side of P's lower leg just below the knee. T's right forearm lies along the medial side of P's lower leg, elbow against the medial side of P's heel.

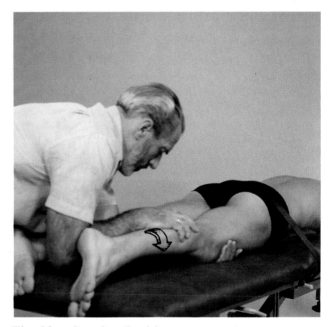

Fig. 92 a. Starting Position.

Procedure: Using this grip, T gradually and fully *medially rotates* at P's hip.

Stimulation of Antagonists: T retains grip, but moves right forearm to lateral side of P's right ankle. T then asks P to move further in the direction of stretching, and resists that movement to stimulate P's antagonists.

Notes: The above procedure assumes that the knee is painful and/or unstable if stressed when flexed, but capable of tolerating stress when extended. For stronger knees, see the previous technique, 6.13.1A, p. 120. For knees unable to tolerate any stress, see the following technique, 6.13.1C, p. 122.

As medial rotation improves with treatment, the hip may successively be abducted more in the starting position.

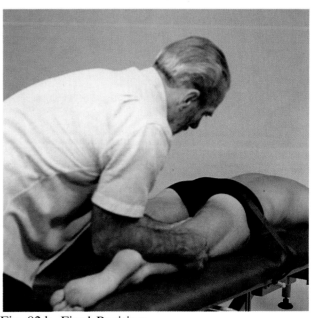

Fig. 92 b. Final Position.

121

6.13.1C. Therapy for the **lateral rotator muscles**. *Alternative technique used, when knee cannot be stressed.*

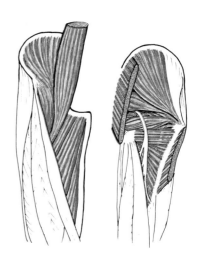

Starting Position: P: Prone; pelvis stabilized with a belt. T: Standing at the right side of the foot of the couch, facing P's head.

Grip: T's right hand dorsally grips P's right trochanter. T's left hand grips the ventral-medial side of P's thigh.

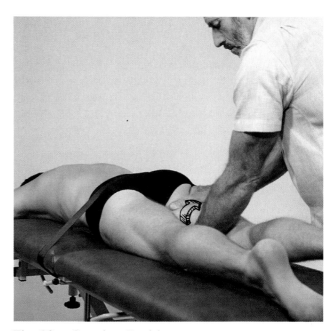

Fig. 93 a. Starting Position.

Procedure: Using this grip, T gradually and fully *medially rotates* at P's hip.

Stimulation of Antagonists: T retains grip . T then asks P to move further in the direction of stretching, and resists that movement to stimulate P's antagonists.

Notes: The above procedure is used when the knee is so painful, unstable or otherwise debilitated that it cannot tolerate external force. For stronger knees, see the preceding two techniques, 6.13.1A and 6.13.1B, pages 120 and 121.

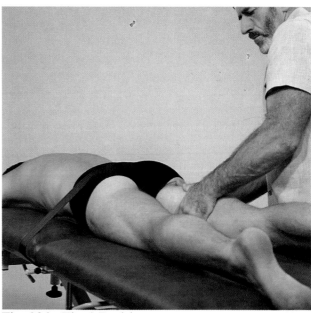

Fig. 93 b. Final Position.

6.14.1A. Therapy for the **medial rotator muscles.** *Knee normal, flexed 90° in treatment.*

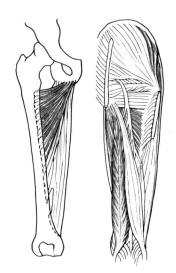

Starting Position: P: Prone; knee flexed approximately 90°; pelvis stabilized with a belt. T: Standing facing P's left side.

Grip: T's right hand grips ventral-lateral side of P's knee and thigh; forearm lies along the lateral side of P's lower leg. T's left hand stabilizes and controls P's sacrum and right ilium.

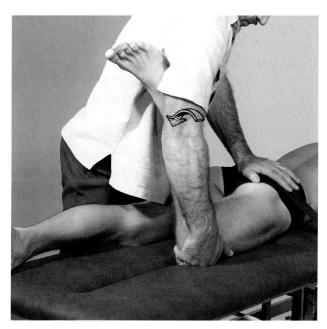

Procedure: Using this grip, T gradually and fully *laterally rotates* at P's hip.

Stimulation of Antagonists: T moves right hand to medial side of P's right leg just proximal to the ankle. T then asks P to move further in the direction of stretching, and resists that movement to stimulate P's antagonists.

Notes: As lateral rotation improves with successive treatments, the abduction at the hip should be increased in the starting position.

This procedure assumes a normal knee capable of tolerating stress when flexed.
In some cases, the knee may be so painful and/or unstable that stress should not be applied to a flexed knee, or not at all to the knee. T must then alter grip and procedure accordingly. See the following two therapy techniques, 6.14.1B and 6.14.1C, pages 124 and 125.

Fig. 94 a. Starting Position.

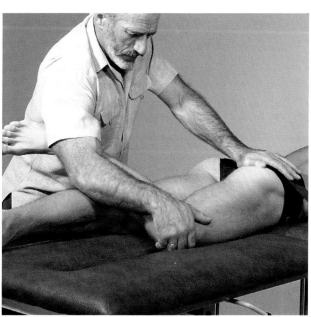

Fig. 94 b. Final Position.

6.14.1B. Therapy for the **medial rotator muscles.** *Alternative technique, used when knee tolerates stress only when extended.*

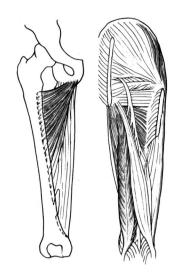

Starting Position: P: Prone; pelvis stabilized with a belt. T: Standing at P's right side facing obliquely towards P.

Grip: T's right hand grips ventral side of P's thigh just above the knee, and T's left hand grips dorsal side of P's lower leg just below the knee. T's left forearm lies along the dorsal-lateral side of P's lower leg, elbow against the lateral side of P's heel.

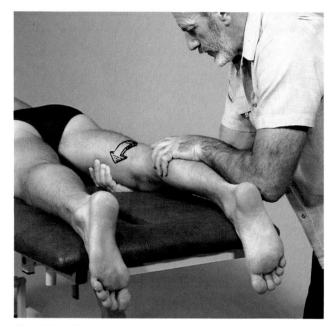

Fig. 95 a. Starting Position.

Procedure: Using this grip, T gradually and fully *laterally rotates* at P's hip.

Stimulation of Antagonists: T retains grip, but moves left forearm to medial side of P's right ankle. T then asks P to move further in the direction of stretching, and resists that movement to stimulate P's antagonists.

Notes: As lateral rotation improves with successive treatment, abduction at the hip should be increased in the starting position.

This procedure assumes that the knee is painful and/or unstable if stressed when flexed, but capable of tolerating stress when extended. For stronger knees, see the previous technique, 6.14.1A, p. 123. For knees unable to tolerate any stress, see the following technique, 6.14.1C, p. 125.

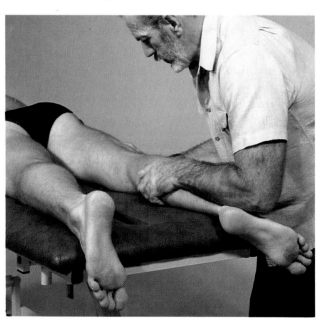

Fig. 95 b. Final Position.

6.14.1C. Therapy for the **medial rotator muscles.** *Alternative technique used, when knee cannot be stressed.*

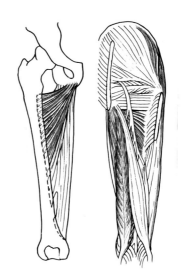

Starting Position: P: Prone; leg slightly abducted to permit grip; pelvis stabilized with a belt. T: Standing at the right side of the foot of the couch, facing P's head.

Grip: T's right hand grips the ventral-lateral side of P's great trochanter. T's left hand grips the dorsal-medial side of P's thigh just below the ischial tuberosity.

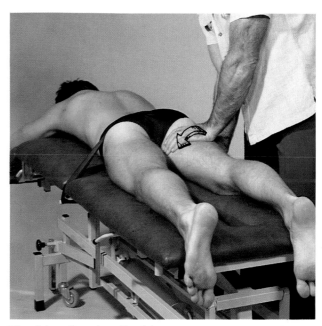

Fig. 96 a. Starting Position.

Procedure: Using this grip, T gradually and fully *laterally rotates* at P's hip.

Stimulation of Antagonists: T retains grip . T then asks P to move further in the direction of stretching, and resists that movement to stimulate P's antagonists.

Note: As lateral rotation improves with successive treatments, abduction at the hip should be increased in the starting position.

This procedure is used when the knee is so painful, unstable or otherwise debilitated that it cannot tolerate external force. For stronger knees, see the preceding two techniques, 6.14.1A and 6.14.1B, pages 123 and 124.

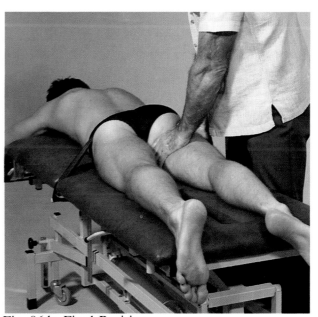

Fig. 96 b. Final Position.

125

7 THE KNEE

7.1 THERAPY GUIDE

The muscles which may restrict movement at the knee are listed in Table 7-1, along with the applicable therapies, indexed by manual section number and page. Muscle actions are listed in Table 7-2. The various restrictions possible are listed in Movement Restriction Table 10.9 (p. 173).

Table 7-1. Restrictions at the knee

SECTION	MOVEMENT RESTRICTED	MUSCLES WHICH MAY RESTRICT MOTION	THERAPY	Number	Page
7.2	*Flexion*	Quadriceps femoris[1]		7.2.1	128
		Tensor fasciae latae[2]		7.2.1	108
7.3	*Flexion and medial rotation (with slight abduction)*	Vastus lateralis, intermedius, and medialis of the quadriceps femoris		7.3.1	129
		Tensor fasciae latae		6.10.2	108
7.4	*Flexion and lateral rotation (with slight adduction)*	Vastus lateralis, intermedius, and medialis of the Quadriceps femoris		7.4.1	130
7.5	*Extension*	Biceps femoris, short head		7.6.1	131
		Plantaris		8.5.1-8.5.3	141-143
		Gastrocnemius		8.5.1	141
		Popliteus		7.7.1	132
7.6	*Extension and medial rotation*	Biceps femoris short head		7.6.1	131
		long head[3]		6.2.1	94
7.7	*Extension and lateral rotation*	Popliteus		7.7.1	132
		Semitendinosus, Semimembranosus, and gracilis[3]		6.2.1	94

NOTES: 1. Restricts when hip is extended or hyperextended.

2. Restricts during extension, adduction and lateral rotation at hip. If the lower leg is medially rotated at the knee, this restriction may increase.

3. May restrict when hip is flexed.

Table 7-2. Actions of muscles which may restrict movement at the knee.

MUSCLE	ACTION
Muscles of the buttocks Tensor fascia latae	Extends and laterally rotates at knee. Abducts, flexes and medially rotates at hip.
Muscles of the thigh Quadriceps femoris	Extends at knee. Rectus femoris also flexes at hip.
Biceps femoris	Long head[1]: Flexes and laterally rotates at knee. Extends, laterally rotates and adducts at hip. Short head: Flexes and laterally rotates at knee.
Gracilis[1]	Adducts at hip. Flexes and laterally rotates when hip is extended. Extends and medially rotates when hip is maximally flexed. Flexes and medially rotates at knee.
Semitendinosus[1]	Flexes and medially rotates at knee. Extends, adducts and medially rotates at hip.
Semimembranosus[1]	Flexes and medially rotates at knee. Extends, adducts and medially rotates at hip.
Muscles of the leg Popliteus	Flexes and medially rotates at knee.
Plantaris	Flexes at knee. Plantar flexes at ankle.
Gastrocnemius	Flexes at knee. Plantar flexes at ankle.

NOTE: 1. Can restrict at knee when hip is flexed.

7.2.1. Therapy for the **quadriceps (vastus lateralis, vastus intermedius** and **vastus medialis).** *Muscle markedly shortened.*

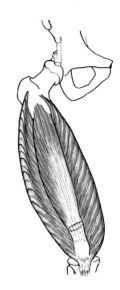

Starting Position: P: Sitting; with lower legs over end of couch; thighs stabilized with a belt; T: Standing between P's legs, facing the medial side of P's right leg.

Grip: T's left hand grips ventral side of P's lower leg just above the ankle. T's right hand lies on the ventral side of P's thigh, for stability of flexing. (If P is very strong, then T may use both hands to grip P's lower leg just above the ankle).

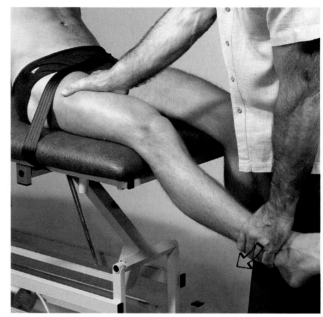

Fig. 97 a. Starting Position.

Procedure: Using this grip, T gradually *flexes* P's knee.

Stimulation of Antagonists: T retains grip. T then asks P to move further in the direction of stretching, and resists that movement to stimulate P's antagonists.

Notes: T should continuously check knee joint for normal glide during treatment.

This procedure may also include medial or lateral rotation at the knee, to stretch the **quadriceps** fully in the position of maximum restriction.

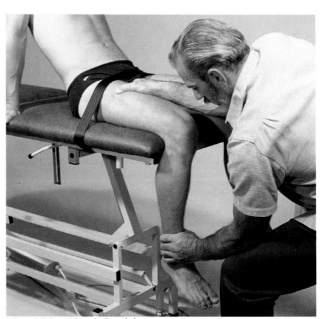

Fig. 97 b. Final Position.

128

7.3.1. Therapy for the **quadriceps (vastus lateralis, vastus intermedius** and **vastus medialis).**

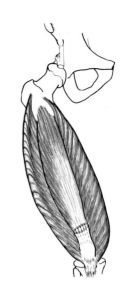

Starting Position: P: Supine; hip and knee flexed approximately 90° (or more, depending on the degree of shortening of the **quadriceps**). T: Standing facing P's leg.

Grip: T's right hand grips the proximal part of P's foot and ankle (or around the ventral-medial side of the lower leg, just proximal to the ankle). T's left hand supports P's knee.

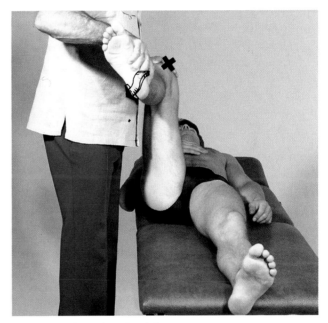

Fig. 98 a. Starting Position.

Procedure: Using this grip, T gradually and fully *flexes*, *abducts* and *medially rotates* at P's knee.

Stimulation of Antagonists: T retains grip. T then asks P to move further in the direction of stretching, and resists that movement to stimulate P's antagonists.

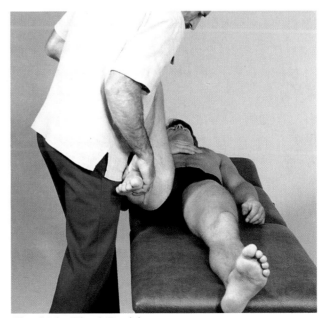

Fig. 98 b. Final Position.

7.4.1. Therapy for the **quadriceps (vastus medialis, vastus intermedius** and **vastus lateralis).**

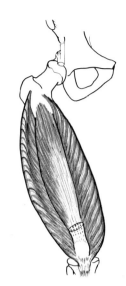

Starting Position: P: Supine; hip and knee flexed approximately 90° (or more, depending on the degree of shortening of the **quadriceps**). T: Standing facing P's leg.

Grip: T's right hand grips around P's right heel from the medial side. T's left hand supports P's knee.

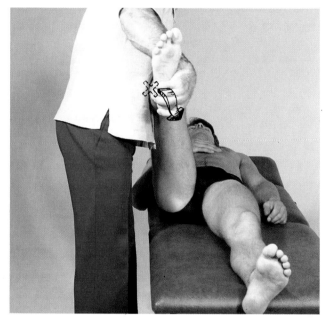

Fig. 99 a. Starting Position.

Procedure: Using this grip, T gradually and fully *flexes*, *adducts* and *laterally rotates* at P's knee.

Stimulation of Antagonists: T moves right forearm to along lateral side of P's right foot, gripping medial side of heel. T then asks P to move further in the direction of stretching, and resists that movement to stimulate P's antagonists.

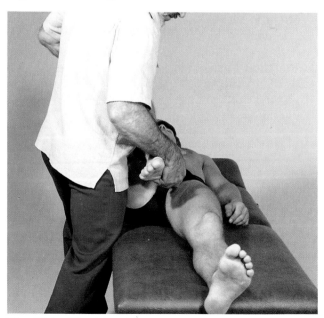

Fig. 99 b. Final Position.

7.6.1. Therapy for the **biceps femoris, short head**.

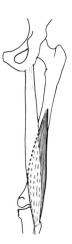

Starting Position: P: Supine; hip and knee extended with knee resting on cushion fully medially rotated. T: Standing facing the lateral side of P's leg.

Grip: T's right hand grips lateral side of P's heel. T's left hand stabilizes P's thigh just above the knee.

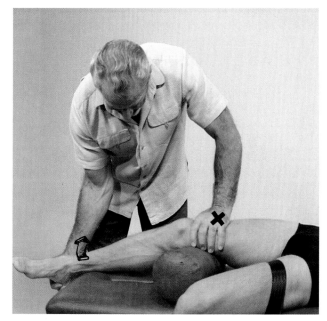

Fig. 100 a. Starting Position.

Procedure: Maintaining this grip, T gradually and fully *medially rotates* and *extends* at P's knee.

Stimulation of Antagonists: T retains grip. T then asks P to move further in the direction of stretching, and resists that movement to stimulate P's antagonists.

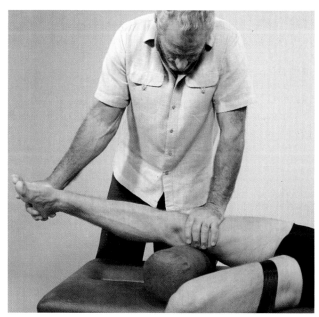

Fig. 100 b. Final Position.

7.7.1.   Therapy for the **popliteus**.

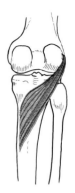

Starting Position: P: Supine; hip and knee extended with knee resting on cushion and fully laterally rotated. T: Standing facing the lateral side of P's lower leg.

Grip: T's right hand grips medial side of P's heel (so that T's forearm and wrist lie against the medial side of P's foot). T's left hand stabilizes P's thigh just above the knee.

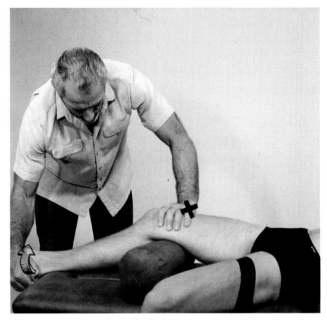

Fig. 101 a. Starting Position.

Procedure: Using this grip, T gradually and fully *laterally rotates* and *extends* at P's knee.

Stimulation of Antagonists: T retains grip. T then asks P to move further in the direction of stretching, and resists that movement to stimulate P's antagonists.

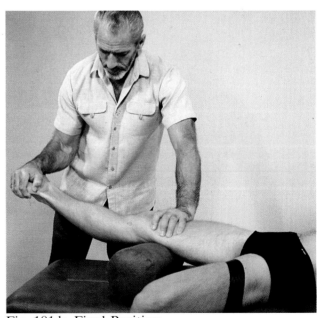

Fig. 101 b. Final Position.

132

8 THE ANKLE

8.1 THERAPY GUIDE

The muscles which may restrict movement at the ankle are listed in Table 8-1, along with the applicable therapies, indexed by manual section number and page. Muscle actions are listed in Table 8-2. The various restrictions possible are listed in Movement Restriction Table 10.10 (p.174).

Table 8.1 Restrictions at the ankle

SECTION	MOVEMENT RESTRICTED	RESTRICTING MUSCLE(S)	THERAPY	Number	Page
8.2	*Plantar flexion*	Tibialis anterior		8.2.1	135
		Extensor hallucis longus		8.2.2	136-137
		Extensor digitorum longus		8.2.3	138-139
		Peroneus tertius		8.2.4	140
8.3	*Plantar flexion and inversion (supination) of foot*	Peroneus tertius		8.2.4	140
		Extensor digitorum longus		8.2.3	138-139
8.4	*Plantar flexion and eversion (pronation) of foot*	Tibialis anterior		8.2.1	135
		Extensor hallucis longus		8.2.2	136-137
8.5	*Dorsal flexion*	Gastrocnemius, plantaris and soleus		8.5.1	141
		Gastrocnemius, lateral head, and plantaris		8.5.2	142
		Gastrocnemius, medial head, and plantaris		8.5.3	143
		Soleus		8.5.4	144-145
		Tibialis posterior		8.5.5	146
		Peroneus longus and brevis		8.5.6	147
		Flexor hallucis longus[2]		9.3.2	154
		Flexor digitorum longus[2]		9.3.4	156
8.6	*Dorsal flexion and inversion (supination) of foot*	Peroneus longus and brevis		8.5.6	147
		Gastrocnemius, lateral head[1]		8.5.1, 8.5.2	141-142
8.7	*Dorsal flexion and eversion (pronation) of foot*	Tibialis posterior		8.5.5	146
		Gastrocnemius, medial head[1]		8.5.1, 8.5.3	141, 143

NOTE: 1. May restrict at ankle with knee extended
       2. May restrict at ankle with toes extended

TABLE 8.2 Actions of muscles which may restrict movements at the ankle.

MUSCLE	ACTION
Tibialis anterior	Dorsal flexes at ankle. Inverts (supinates) the foot.
Extensor hallucis longus	Dorsal flexes at ankle. Inverts (supinates) foot.
Extensor digitorum longus	Dorsal flexes at ankle. Extends at DIP, PIP and MTP joints.
Peroneus tertius	Dorsal flexes at ankle. Everts (pronates) foot.
Peroneus longus and brevis	Plantar flex at ankle. Evert (pronate) foot.
Flexor hallucis longus	Plantar flexes at ankle. Flexes at IP and MTP joints of great toe. Inverts (supinates) foot.
Flexor digitorum longus	Plantar flexes at ankle. Flexes at MTP, PIP and DIP joints. Inverts (supinates) foot.
Gastrocnemius	Flexes at knee. Plantar flexes at ankle.
Plantaris	Flexes at knee. Plantar flexes at ankle.
Soleus	Plantar flexes at ankle.
Tibialis posterior	Plantar flexes at ankle. Inverts (supinates) foot. Adducts foot.

Joint abbreviations:

DIP Distal-interphalangeal
IP   Interphalangeal
MTP Metatarsal-phalangeal
PIP Proximal-interphalangeal

8.2.1.   Therapy for the **tibialis anterior**.

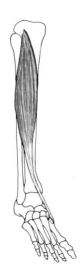

Starting Position: P: Supine; ankle over end of the couch. (It is easier to glide the talus against the tibia if P's heel is held against the couch. However, if P has pain in the heel or subtalar joints, this starting position cannot be used); foot fully everted (pronated). T: Standing facing the lateral side of P's lower leg.

Grip: T's right hand grips P's instep, from the cuneiform bones down through the toes, with fingers curling around the medial side of the foot onto the sole. T's left hand stabilizes P's lower leg just below the knee.

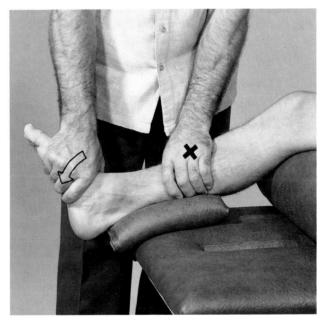

Fig. 102 a. Starting Position.

Procedure: Using this grip, T gradually and fully *plantar flexes* at P's ankle.

Stimulation of Antagonists: T retains grip. T then asks P to move further in the direction of stretching, and resists that movement to stimulate P's antagonists.

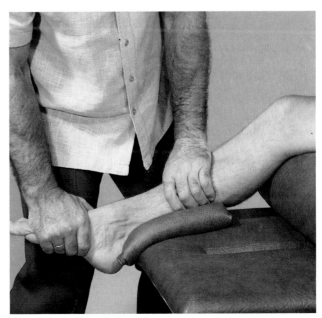

Fig. 102 b. Final Position.

8.2.2A.   Therapy for the **extensor hallucis longus**.

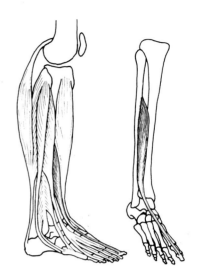

Starting Position: P: Supine; ankle dorsally flexed and over end of couch; lower leg stabilized with a belt. T: Standing facing the lateral side of P's foot.

Grip: T's left hand grips the middle of P's foot from the medial side, with fingers plantar on foot, covering the MTP joints. T's right hand stabilizes P's great toe by gripping the distal phalanx and holding the IP and MTP joints fully flexed.

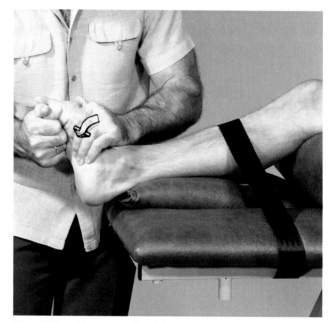

Fig. 103 a. Starting Position.

Procedure: Using this grip, T gradually and fully *plantar flexes* at P's ankle while *everting* (pronating) P's foot.

Stimulation of Antagonists: T retains grip. T then asks P to move further in the direction of stretching, and resists that movement to stimulate P's antagonists.

Note: This procedure may also be performed with one hand, see the following technique, therapy 8.2.2B, p. 137.

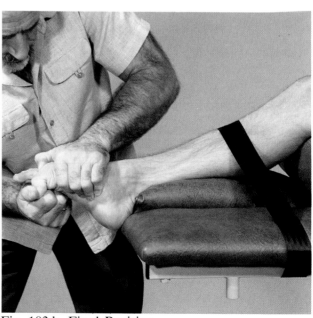

Fig. 103 b. Final Position.

8.2.2B. Therapy for the **extensor hallucis longus**. *Alternative one-hand grip.*

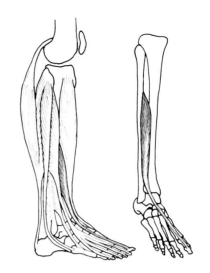

Starting Position: P: Supine; ankle dorsally flexed and held over the end of the couch; lower leg stabilized with a belt. T: Standing facing the lateral side of P's foot.

Grip: T's left hand stabilizes P's lower leg. T's right hand grips around P's great toe over the MTP joint and fully flexes at the IP and MTP joints.

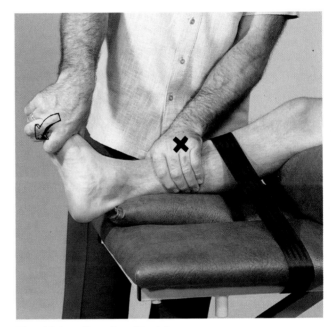

Fig. 104 a. Starting Position.

Procedure: Using this grip, T gradually and fully *plantar flexes* at P's ankle while *everting* (pronating) P's foot.

Stimulation of Antagonists: T retains grip. T then asks P to move further in the direction of stretching, and resists that movement to stimulate P's antagonists.

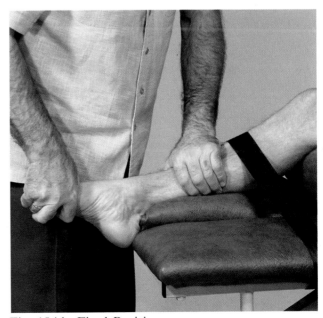

Fig. 104 b. Final Position.

8.2.3A. Therapy for the **extensor digitorum longus.** *Toes simultaneously.*

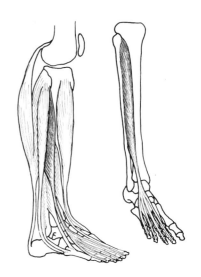

Starting Position: P: Supine; ankle dorsally flexed and over end of couch; lower leg stabilized with a belt. T: Standing facing the lateral side of P's foot.

Grip: T's left hand grips the middle of the medial/plantar side of P's foot. T's right hand stabilizes P's 2nd through 5th toes by gripping them from the dorsal side and holding them fully flexed at the DIP, PIP and MTP joints.

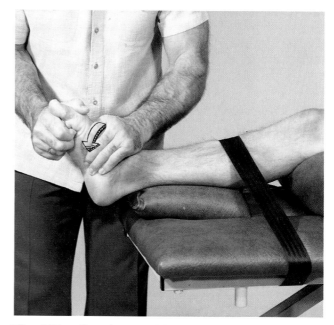

Fig. 105 a. Starting Position.

Procedure: Using this grip, T gradually and fully *plantar flexes* at P's ankle.

Stimulation of Antagonists: T retains grip. T then asks P to move further in the direction of stretching, and resists that movement to stimulate P's antagonists.

Note: The toes may be treated individually, see the following technique, therapy 8.2.3B, p. 139.

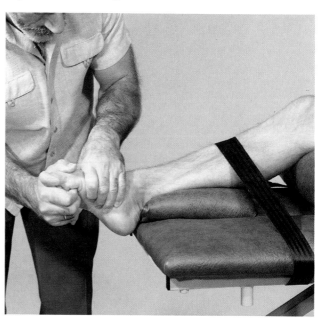

Fig. 105 b. Final Position.

8.2.3B. Therapy for the **extensor digitorum longus.** *Toes individually.*

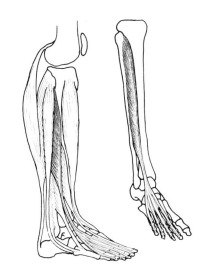

Starting Position: P: Supine; ankle dorsally flexed and over end of couch; lower leg stabilized with a belt just below the patella. T: Standing at foot of couch facing the lateral side of P's foot.

Grip: T's left hand grips instep of P's foot. T's right hand stabilizes one of the lateral toes (2nd shown here) by fully flexing it at the MTP and DIP joints.

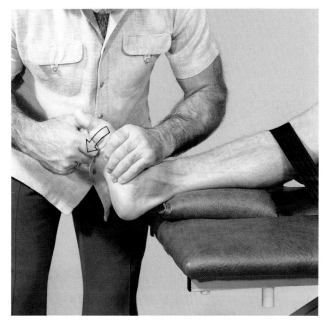

Fig. 106 a. Starting Position.

Procedure: Using this grip, T gradually and fully *plantar flexes* at P's ankle.

Stimulation of Antagonists: T retains grip. T then asks P to move further in the direction of stretching, and resists that movement to stimulate P's antagonists.

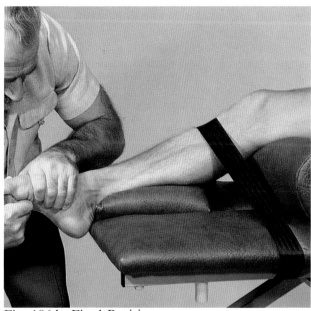

Fig. 106 b. Final Position.

8.2.4.   Therapy for the **peroneus tertius**.

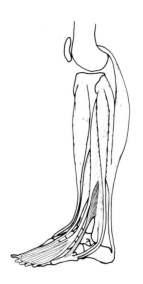

Starting Position: P: Supine; ankle dorsally flexed and over end of couch; lower leg is stabilized with a belt. T: Standing facing the medial side of P's right foot.

Grip: T's left hand grips over instep P's foot, including the base of the 5th metatarsal, and holds the foot fully inverted (supinated). T's right hand grips P's lower leg just above the ankle, stabilizing it to the couch.

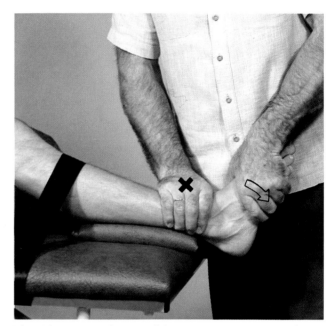

Fig. 107 a. Starting Position.

Procedure: Using this grip, T gradually and fully *plantar flexes* at P's ankle.

Stimulation of Antagonists: T retains grip. T then asks P to move further in the direction of stretching, and resists that movement to stimulate P's antagonists.

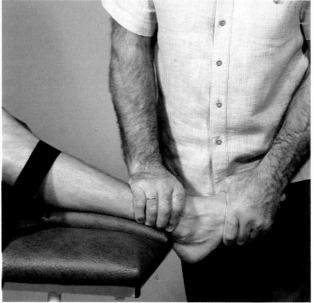

Fig. 107 b. Final Position.

8.5.1. Therapy for the **gastrocnemius, plantaris** and **soleus**.

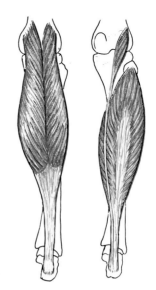

Starting Position: P: Standing, leaning forward against a wall; left leg forward, knee and hip flexed; right leg extended rearwards, toes and ball of foot on floor. T: Standing to the side of, and behind, P's right leg.

Grip: T's right hand grips the ventral side of P's knee from the dorsal-medial aspect. T's left hand grips dorsal side of P's lower leg.

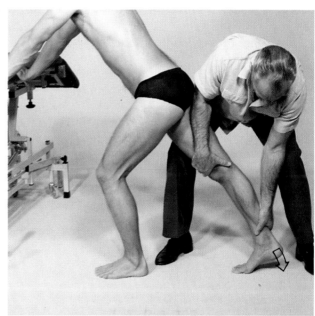

Fig. 108 a. Starting Position.

Procedure: Using this grip, T (with P's help) gradually presses P's heel to the floor to *dorsally flex* at P's ankle.

Stimulation of Antagonists: P rocks back on right heel, retaining ankle dorsal flexion so ball of foot rises from floor. T places right hand on dorsal side of P's foot. T then asks P to move his foot further in the direction of stretching, and T resists that movement to stimulate P's antagonists.

Note: To further increase dorsal flexion at ankle, move P's foot further back.

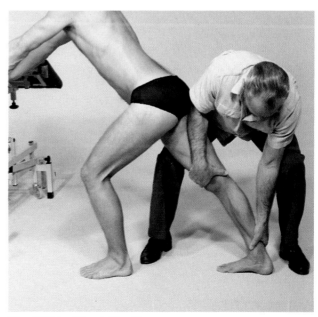

Fig. 108 b. Final Position.

Therapy for the **gastrocnemius, lateral head**.

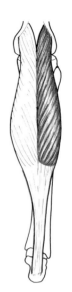

Starting Position: P: Standing, leaning forward obliquely against a wall; left leg forward, knee slightly flexed; right leg extended rearwards, toes and ball of foot on floor, heel and instep on wedge to supinate foot. T: Standing behind P, facing the medial-dorsal side of P's leg.

Grip: T's left hand grips the ventral side of P's knee from the dorsal-lateral aspect. T's right hand grips dorsal side of P's lower leg.

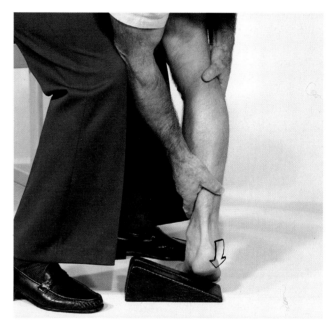

Fig. 109 a. Starting Position.

Procedure: Using this grip, T (with P's help) gradually presses P's heel to the floor (in the *varus* position) to *dorsally flex* at P's ankle.

Stimulation of Antagonists: P rocks back on right heel, retaining ankle dorsal flexion and supination. T places left hand on dorsal-medial side of P's foot. T then asks P to move further in the direction of stretching, and resists that movement to stimulate P's antagonists.

Note: The less the angle between the rearward leg and the floor, the greater the stretching achieved.

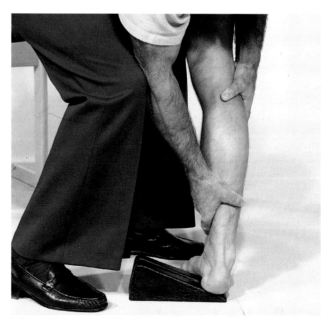

Fig. 109 b. Final Position.

8.5.3. Therapy for the **gastrocnemius, medial head** and the **plantaris**.

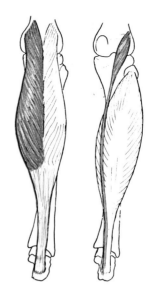

Starting Position: P: Standing, leaning forward obliquely against a wall; left leg forward, knee slightly flexed; right leg extended rearwards, toes and ball of foot on floor, heel and lateral side of sole on wedge to pronate foot. T: Standing behind P, facing the lateral-dorsal side of P's leg.

Grip: T's right hand grips the ventral side of P's knee from the dorsal-medial aspect. T's left hand grips the dorsal side of P's lower leg, just below the knee.

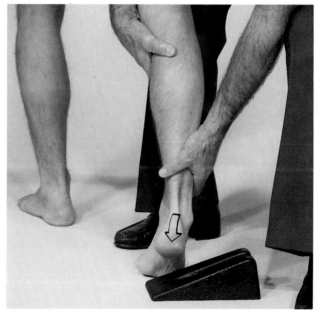

Fig. 110 a. Starting Position.

Procedure: Using this grip, T (with P's help) gradually presses P's heel to the floor (with foot in the *valgus* position) to *dorsally flex* at the ankle.

Stimulation of Antagonists: P rocks back on right heel, retaining ankle dorsal flexion and pronation. T places right hand on lateral-dorsal side of P's foot. T then asks P to move further in the direction of stretching, and resists that movement to stimulate P's antagonists.

Note: The less the angle between the rearward leg and the floor, the greater the stretching.

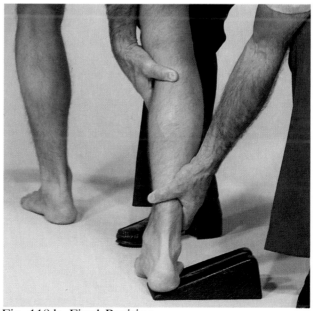

Fig. 110 b. Final Position.

8.5.4A. Therapy for the **soleus**.

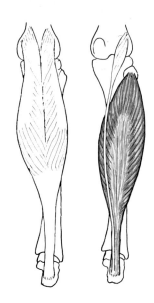

Starting Position: P: Standing, leaning forward obliquely against a wall; left leg forward, knee slightly flexed; right hip and knee extended with heel stabilized on the floor. T: Standing behind P, facing the lateral/dorsal side of P's leg.

Grip: T's right hand grips the dorsal side of P's leg just distal to the knee. T's left hand grips P's heel and stabilizes it against the floor.

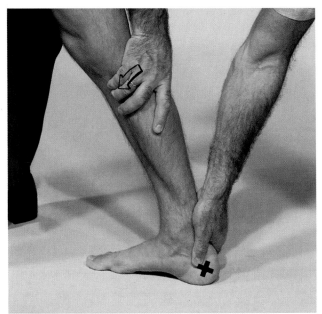

Fig. 111 a. Starting Position.

Procedure: Using this grip, T (with P's help) gradually *flexes* P's right knee while keeping the heel against the floor to produce full *dorsal flexion* at the ankle.

Stimulation of Antagonists: P rocks back on right heel, retaining ankle dorsal flexion and knee flexion. T places right hand on dorsal side of P's foot. T then asks P to move further in the direction of stretching, and resists that movement to stimulate P's antagonists.

Note: If P's foot is small and/or might deform, or otherwise P cannot tolerate erect position with foot loaded, treatment may be performed with P prone, see therapy 8.5.4B, p. 145.

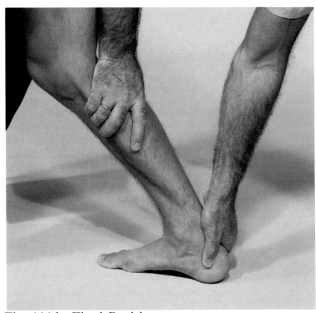

Fig. 111 b. Final Position.

8.5.4B. Therapy for the **soleus.** *Alternative, with P prone.*

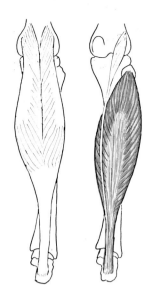

Starting Position: P: Prone; P's knee flexed approximately 90°; T: Standing, facing the lateral side of P's lower leg.

Grip: T's left hand stabilizes P's heel, forearm along the sole of P's foot. T's right hand grips instep from the dorsal-medial side. To increase stability and/or force applied, P's foot may be supported against T's chest.

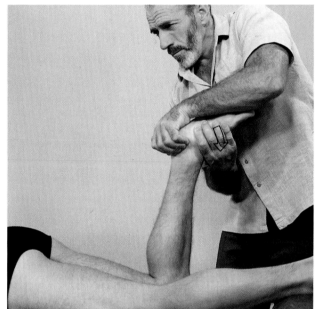

Fig. 112 a. Starting Position.

Procedure: Using this grip, T gradually and fully *dorsal flexes* at P's ankle.

Stimulation of Antagonists: T retains grip. T then asks P to move further in the direction of stretching, and resists that movement to stimulate P's antagonists.

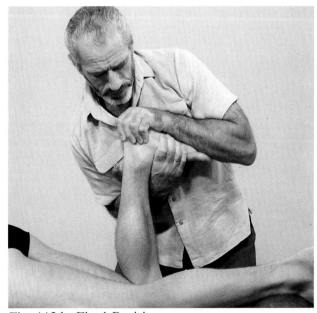

Fig. 112 b. Final Position.

145

8.5.5.   Therapy for the **tibialis posterior**.

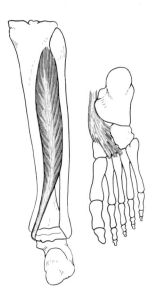

Starting Position: P: Prone; knee flexed approximately 90°. T: Standing facing the lateral side of P's lower leg.

Grip: T's left hand grips the plantar side of P's foot, with fingers around the medial side (including the navicular bone), and holds the foot fully everted (pronated) and abducted. T's right hand stabilizes P's leg by gripping the medial side of the lower leg just proximal to the ankle.

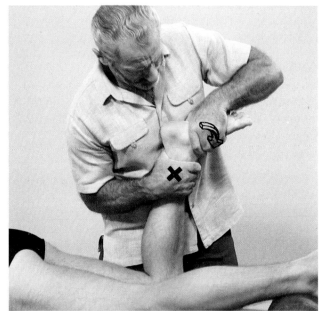

Fig. 113 a. Starting Position.

Procedure: Using this grip, T gradually and fully *dorsal flexes* at P's ankle.

Stimulation of Antagonists: T moves left hand to lateral-dorsal side of P's foot. T then asks P to move further in the direction of stretching, and resists that movement to stimulate P's antagonists.

Note: This technique may also be used for treating restricted dorsal flexion at the ankle *and* restricted eversion of the foot.

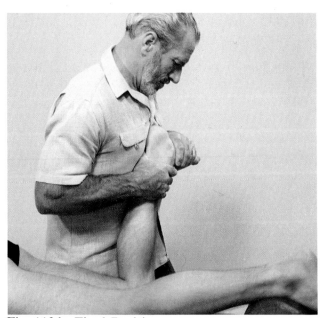

Fig. 113 b. Final Position.

146

8.5.6. Therapy for the **peroneus longus and brevis**.

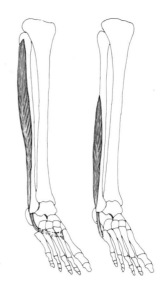

Starting Position: P: Prone; knee flexed approximately 90°. T: Standing facing the lateral side of P's lower leg.

Grip: T's left hand grips plantar-lateral side of P's foot (including the cuboid bone). T's right hand stabilizes P's leg by gripping the medial side of the lower leg just above the ankle. T holds P's foot fully inverted (supinated). To increase stability, P's foot may be supported against T's abdomen or chest.

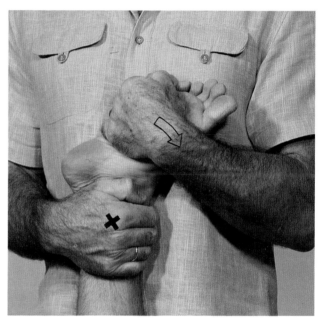

Fig. 114 a. Starting Position.

Procedure: Using this grip, T gradually and fully *dorsal flexes* at P's ankle.

Stimulation of Antagonists: T moves left hand to dorsal-lateral side of P's foot. T then asks P to move further in the direction of stretching, and resists that movement to stimulate P's antagonists.

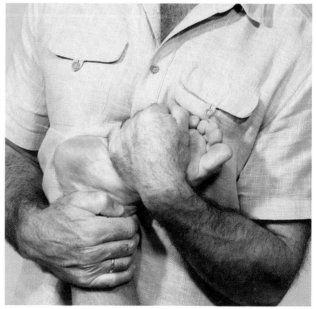

Fig. 114 b. Final Position.

9   THE TOES

9.1   THERAPY GUIDE

The muscles which may restrict movement at the joints of the toes are listed in Table 9-1, along with the applicable therapies, indexed by manual section numer and page. Muscle actions are listed in Table 9-2.

The various restrictions possible are listed in Movement Restriction Table 10.11 (p. 175).

TABLE 9.1   Restrictions at the joints of the toes

Section	MOVEMENT RESTRICTED	RESTRICTING MUSCLE(S)	THERAPY	Number	Page
9.2	*Flexion*	Extensor hallucis brevis		**9.2.1**	150
		Extensor hallucis longus		**8.2.2**	136-137
		Extensor digitorum brevis		**9.2.2**	151-152
		Extensor digitorum longus		**8.2.3**	138-139
9.3	Extension	Flexor hallucis brevis		**9.3.1**	153
		Flexor hallucis longus		**9.3.2**	154
		Flexor digitorum brevis		**9.3.3**	155
		Flexor digitorum longus		**9.3.4**	156
		Lumbricales		**9.3.5**	157
		Interossei dorsales		**9.6.1**	161
		Plantares		**9.7.1**	162
9.4	*Abduction at MTP joint of great toe*	Adductor hallucis		**9.4.1**	158
		Flexor hallucis brevis		**9.3.1**	153
9.5	*Adduction at MTP joint of great toe[1]*	Abductor hallucis		**9.5.1**	159
		Flexor hallucis brevis, tibial part		**9.5.2**	160
9.6	*Lateral movement of lateral toes towards fibula*	Interossei plantares and Interosseus dorsales I		**9.6.1**	161
9.7	*Medial movement of lateral toes towards tibia*	Interossei dorsales II, III and IV, Abductor digiti minimi, and flexor digiti minimi brevis		**9.7.1**	162

NOTE: 1.   Very uncommon

TABLE 9.2 Actions of muscles which may restrict movements at the joints.

MUSCLE	ACTION
Muscles of the leg	
Extensor hallucis longus	Dorsal flexes at ankle. Inverts (supinates) foot. Extends at IP and MTP joints.
Extensor digitorum longus	Dorsal flexes at ankle. Extends at DIP, PIP and MTP joints.
Flexor hallucis longus	Flexes at IP and MTP joints of great toe. Plantar flexes at ankle. Inverts (supinates) foot.
Flexor digitorum longus	Flexes at MTP, PIP and DIP joints. Plantar flexes ankle. Inverts (supinates) foot.
Muscles of the foot	
Extensor hallucis brevis	Extends at MTP joint of great toe.
Flexor hallucis brevis	Lateral part adducts and flexes at MTP joint, medial part abducts and flexes at MTP joint of great toe.
Extensor digitorum brevis	Extends at the PIP and MTP joints.
Flexor digitorum brevis	Flexes at MTP and PIP joints.
Lumbricales	Extends at DIP and PIP joints. Flex at MTP joints.
Interossei plantares	Move 3rd, 4th and 5th toes towards tibia. Flex at MTP joints, and extend at DIP and PIP joints.
Interossei dorsales	Extend at DIP and PIP joints. Flex at MTP joints. I moves 2nd toe medially towards tibia. II, III and IV move 2nd, 3rd and 4th toes laterally towards fibula.
Adductor hallucis	Adducts and flexes at MTP joint of great toe.
Abductor hallucis	Abducts and flexes at MTP joint of great toe.
Abductor digiti minimi	Flexes and abducts little toe laterally towards fibula.
Flexor digiti minimi brevis	Flexes and abducts little toe laterally towards fibula.

NOTES: 1. Joint abbrevaiation:DIP - Distal-interphalangeal, IP - Interphalangeal, MTP - Metatarsalphalangeal, PIP - Proximal-interphalangeal.
2. Terms abduct, adduct, medial and lateral are sometimes ambiguous when applied to the toes. Therefor, for clarity, terms towards the fibula, towards the tibia, fibular and tibial are used whenever other anatomical terms may mislead.

9.2.1. Therapy for the **extensor hallucis brevis**.

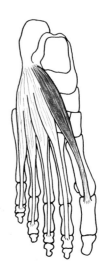

Starting Position: P: Supine; ankle dorsally flexed. T: Standing facing the lateral side of P's foot.

Grip: T's right hand grips P's great toe near the MTP-joint. T's left hand stabilizes P's forefoot from the medial/plantar side.

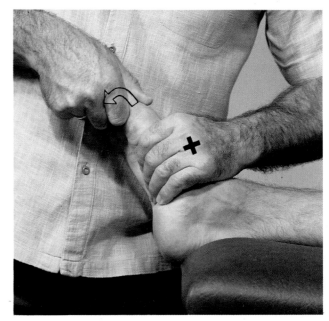

Fig. 115 a. Starting Position.

Procedure: Using this grip, T applies traction while gradually and fully *flexing* at the MTP-joint of the great toe.

Stimulation of Antagonists: T retains grip. T then asks P to move further in the direction of stretching, and resists that movement to stimulate P's antagonists.

Note: Continuously check for normal MTP joint glide during treatment.

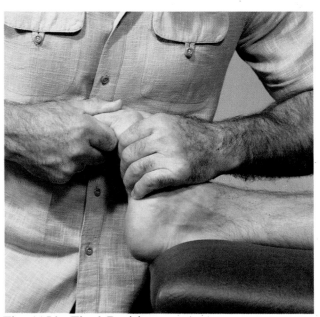

Fig. 115 b. Final Position.

9.2.2A. Therapy for the **extensor digitorum brevis**. *Toes individually.*

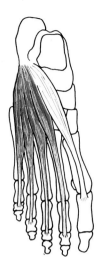

Starting Position: P: Supine; ankle dorsally flexed to prevent interference from the **extensor digitorum longus**. (If P's **gastrocnemius** is shortened, the knee must be flexed to permit full dorsal flexion at the ankle). T: Standing at foot of couch facing the lateral side of P's right foot.

Grip: T's right hand grips one of lateral toes (2nd toe illustrated), thumb on dorsal side with index finger on plantar side, and holds the PIP joint fully flexed. T's left hand stabilizes P's foot by gripping instep.

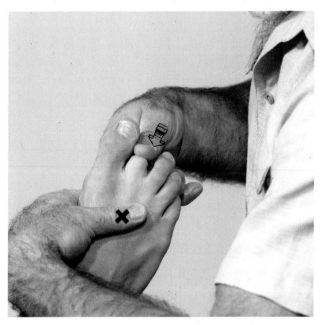

Fig. 116 a. Starting Position.

Procedure: Maintaining this grip, T applies traction at the MTP joint while gradually and fully *flexing* P's the toe.

Stimulation of Antagonists: T retains grip. T then asks P to move further in the direction of stretching, and resists that movement to stimulate P's antagonists.

Note: Continuously check for normal MTP joint glide during treatment.

If all toes are restricted, T may treat toes simultaneously using the following technique, therapy 9.2.2B, p. 152.

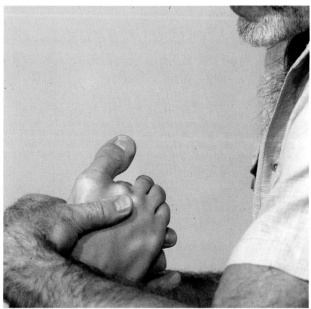

Fig. 116 b. Final Position.

9.2.2B. Therapy for the **extensor digitorum brevis.** *Four lateral toes simultaneously.*

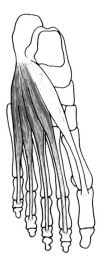

Starting Position: P: Supine; ankle dorsally flexed to prevent interference from the **extensor digitorum longus.** (If P's **gastrocnemius** is shortened, the knee must be flexed to permit full dorsal flexion at the ankle). T: Standing, left side against the lateral side of P's leg, facing the dorsum of P's foot.

Grip: T's right hand grips P's lateral toes near the PIP joints from the dorsal side. T's left hand stabilizes P's foot by gripping the medial- plantar side.

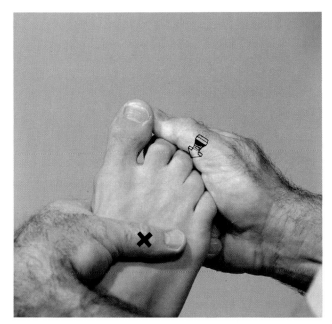

Fig. 117 a. Starting Position.

Procedure: Using this grip, T applies traction at the PIP and MTP joints while gradully and fully *flexing* the toes.

Stimulation of Antagonists: T retains grip. T then asks P to move further in the direction of stretching, and resists that movement to stimulate P's antagonists.

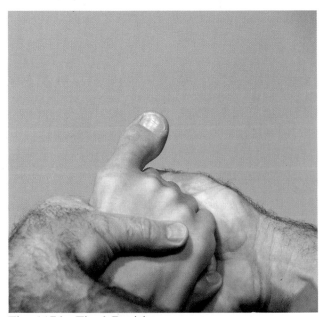

Fig. 117 b. Final Position.

9.3.1. Therapy for the **flexor hallucis brevis**.

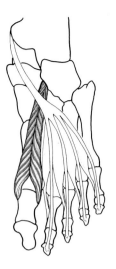

Starting Position: P: Prone; knee flexed approximately 90°; ankle plantar flexed to avoid interference from the **flexor hallucis longus**. T: Standing facing the lateral side of P's foot.

Grip: T's left hand grips P's great toe near the MTP joint. T's right hand stabilizes P's foot by gripping the medial-dorsal side near the MTP joint. To increase stability, P's foot may be supported against T's abdomen or chest.

Procedure: Using this grip, T applies traction at the MTP joint while gradually and fully *extending* the great toe.

Stimulation of Antagonists: T retains grip. T then asks P to move further in the direction of stretching, and resists that movement to stimulate P's antagonists.

Notes: Continuously check for normal MTP joint glide during treatment.

To specifically stretch:

Flexor hallucis brevis, tibial part	See p. 160.
Flexor hallucis brevis, fibular part	See p. 158.

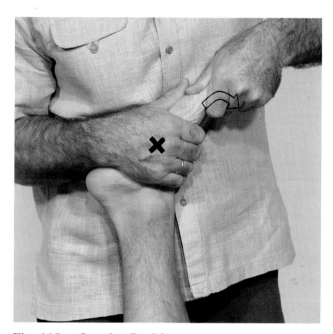

Fig. 118 a. Starting Position.

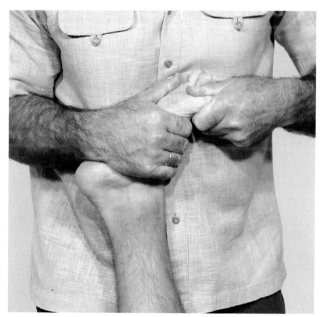

Fig. 118 b. Final Position.

9.3.2. Therapy for the **flexor hallucis longus**.

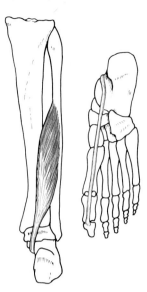

Starting Position: P: Prone; knee flexed approximately 90°; ankle plantar flexed. T: Standing facing the lateral side of P's foot.

Grip: T's left hand stabilizes P's great toe near the MTP joint and fully extends the IP and MTP joints. T's right hand grips P's foot from the plantarmedial side. To increase stability and/or force applied, P's foot may be supported against T's abdomen or chest.

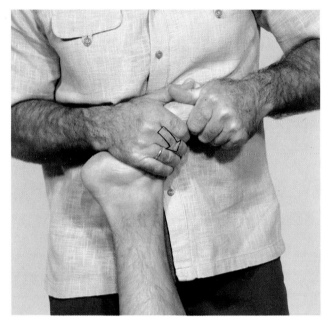

Fig. 119 a. Starting Position.

Procedure: Using this grip, T gradually and fully *dorsal flexes* at P's ankle.

Stimulation of Antagonists: T retains grip. T then asks P to move further in the direction of stretching, and resists that movement to stimulate P's antagonists.

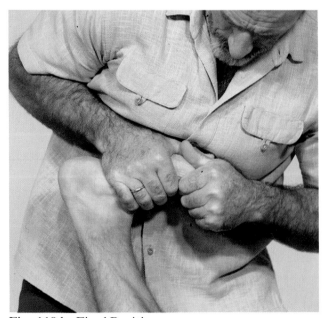

Fig. 119 b. Final Position.

9.3.3. Therapy for the **flexor digitorum brevis**.

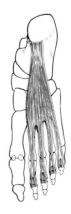

Starting Position: P: Prone; knee flexed approximately 90°; ankle plantar flexed. T: Standing facing the lateral side of P's right foot.

Grip: T's left hand grips near the MTP joint of one of P's lateral toes (2nd toe illustrated). (To obtain a firm grip on the toe, both the DIP and the PIP joints must be extended). T's right hand stabilizes P's foot by gripping the medial-dorsal side. To increase stability, P's foot may be supported against T's abdomen or chest.

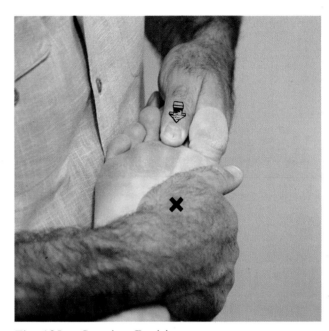

Fig. 120 a. Starting Position.

Procedure: Maintaining this grip, T applies traction at P's MTP joint while T gradually and fully *extends* the toe.

Stimulation of Antagonists: T retains grip. T then asks P to move further in the direction of stretching, and resists that movement to stimulate P's antagonists.

Notes: Continuously check for normal MTP joint glide during treatment.

This technique may be used to treat the toes individually (as shown, for 2nd toe) or to treat two, three or all four lateral toes simultaneously, by accordingly altering grip.

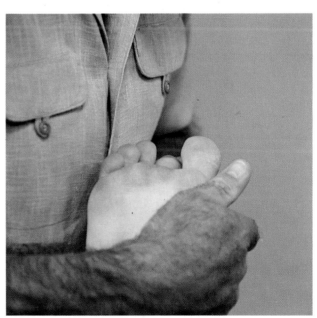

Fig. 120 b. Final Position.

9.3.4. Therapy for the **flexor digitorum longus**.

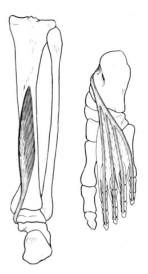

Starting Position: P: Prone; knee flexed approximately 90°; ankle plantar flexed; foot fully everted (pronated). T: Standing facing the lateral side of P's foot.

Grip: T's left hand stabilizes one or more of P's toes by fully extending at the DIP and PIP joints and fully dorsally flexing at the MTP joints. T's right hand grips the plantar-medial side of P's foot. To increase force applied, P's foot may be supported against T's chest.

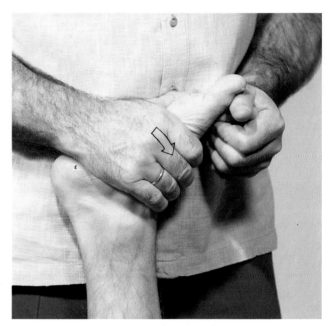

Fig. 121 a. Starting Position.

Procedure: Using this grip, T gradually and fully *dorsal flexes* at P's ankle.

Stimulation of Antagonists: T retains grip. T then asks P to move further in the direction of stretching, and resists that movement to stimulate P's antagonists.

Note: Initial position of toe(s) relative to foot must be carefully maintained as ankle is dorsally flexed.

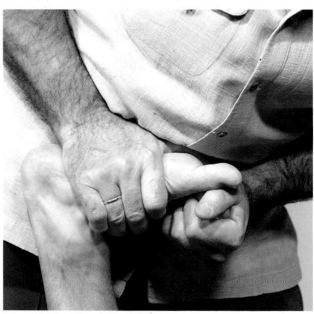

Fig. 121 b. Final Position.

9.3.5.   Therapy for the **lumbricales**.

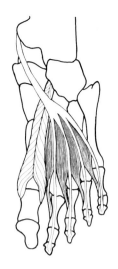

Starting Position: P: Prone; knee flexed approximately 90°; ankle in neutral position. T: Standing facing P's left side.

Grip: T's right hand stabilizes P's lateral toes by fully flexing at the DIP and PIP joints while fully extending at the MTP joints. T's left hand grips around P's foot from plantar side. To increase force applied, P's foot may be supported against T's chest.

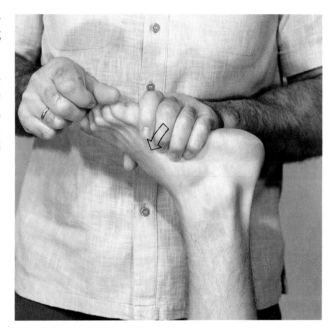

Fig. 122 a. Starting Position.

Procedure: Using this grip, T gradually and fully *dorsally flexes* at P's ankle.

Stimulation of Antagonists: T retains grip. T then asks P to move further in the direction of stretching, and resists that movement to stimulate P's antagonists.

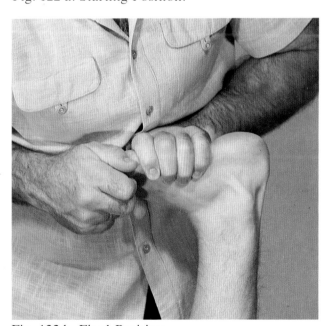

Fig. 122 b. Final Position.

9.4.1. Therapy for the **adductor hallucis** and the flexor hallucis brevis, fibular part.

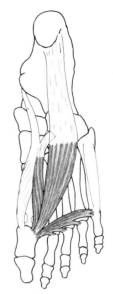

Starting Position: P: Supine; ankle in neutral position. T: Standing facing the medial side of P's foot.

Grip: T's left hand grips P's great toe near the MTP joint. T's right hand stabilizes P's foot at the medial-dorsal side near the MTP joint of the great toe.

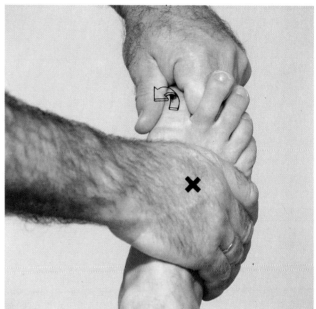

Fig. 123 a. Starting Position.

Procedure: Maintaining this grip, T applies traction at the MTP joint while gradually and fully *abducting, extending* and laterally rotating the great toe (dorsal aspect of the great toe moves in tibial direction).

Stimulation of Antagonists: T retains grip. T then asks P to move further in the direction of stretching, and resists that movement to stimulate P's antagonists.

Notes: Continuously check for normal MTP joint glide during treatment.

This technique may be used for treating hallux valgus.

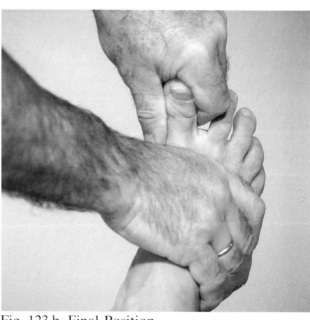

Fig. 123 b. Final Position.

158

9.5.1. Therapy for the **abductor hallucis** and the flexor hallucis brevis, tibial part.

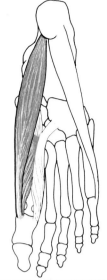

Starting Position: P: Supine; ankle in neutral position. T: Standing facing the lateral side of P's foot.

Grip: T's right hand grips P's great toe near the MTP joint, thumb along the fibular side and flexed index finger along the tibial side. T's left hand stabilizes P's foot at the dorsal-medial side near the MTP joint of the great toe.

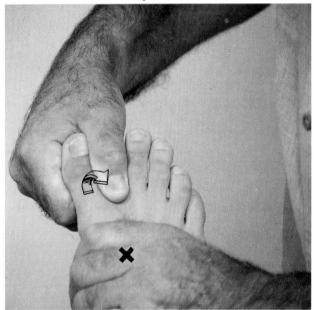

Fig. 124 a. Starting Position.

Procedure: Using this grip, T applies traction at the MTP joint while gradually and fully *adducting, extending* and medially rotating the great toe (dorsal aspect of the great toe moves in fibular direction).

Stimulation of Antagonists: T retains grip. T then asks P to move further in the direction of stretching, and resists that movement to stimulate P's antagonists.

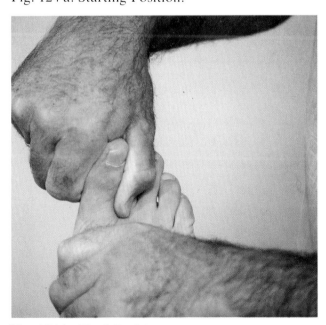

Fig. 124 b. Final Position.

9.5.2. Therapy for the **flexor hallucis brevis, tibial part**

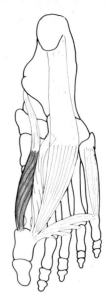

Starting Position: P: Supine; ankle in neutral position. T: Standing facing the lateral side of P's foot.

Grip: T's right hand grips the distal phalanx of P's great toe, thumb along the dorsal side and flexed index finger on the plantar side. T's left hand stabilizes P's foot from the dorsal-medial side near the MTP joint of the great toe.

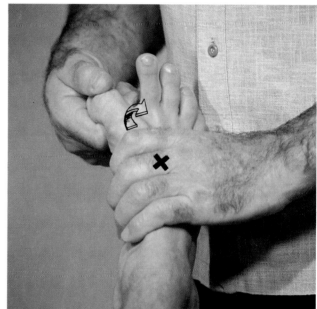

Fig. 125 a. Starting Position.

Procedure: Maintaining this grip, T applies traction at the MTP joint of P's great toe while gradually and fully *extending, adducting* and medially rotating the proximal phalanx, (dorsal aspect of the great toe moves in fibular direction).

Stimulation of Antagonists: T retains grip. T then asks P to move further in the direction of stretching, and resists that movement to stimulate P's antagonists.

Note: Stretching is easier when the entire great toe is gripped. However, the ankle must then be plantar flexed, to relax the flexor hallucis longus.

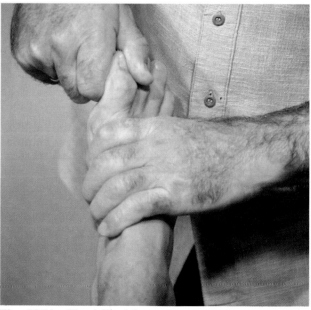

Fig. 125 b. Final Position.

9.6.1. Therapy for the **interossei plantares** and **interosseus dorsalis I**.

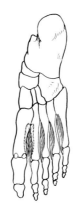

Starting Position: P: Supine; ankle in neutral position. T: Standing facing the lateral side of P's foot.

Grip: T's right hand grips near the MTP joints of P's lateral toes and fully flexes them at the DIP and PIP joints. T's left hand stabilizes P's foot at the dorsal-medial side near the MTP-joints.

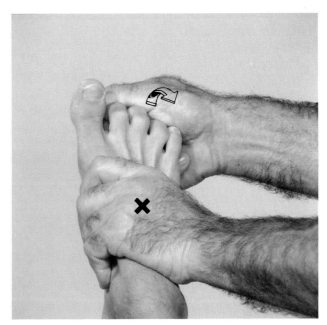

Fig. 126 a. Starting Position.

Procedure: Using this grip, with toes maximally flexed at the DIP and PIP joints, T applies traction at the MTP joints while gradually and fully *dorsal flexing* at the MTP joints and drawing toes *laterally* towards the fibula.

Stimulation of Antagonists: T retains grip. T then asks P to move further in the direction of stretching, and resists that movement to stimulate P's antagonists.

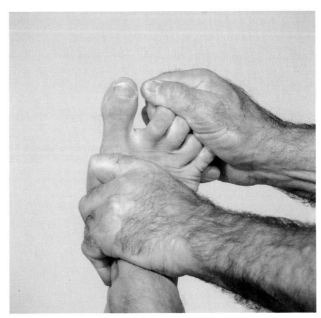

Fig. 126 b. Final Position.

9.7.1. Therapy for the **interossei dorsales II, III and IV, abductor digiti minimi and flexor digiti minimi brevis.**

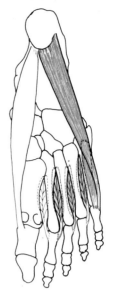

Starting Position: P: Supine; foot in neutral position. T: Standing facing the lateral side of P's foot.

Grip: T's right hand grips near the MTP joints of P's lateral toes, thumb and thenar eminence over the dorsal side and fingers along the plantar side. T's left hand stabilizes P's foot at the dorsal-medial side near the MTP joints. T's right hand then fully flexes the four toes at the DIP and PIP joints.

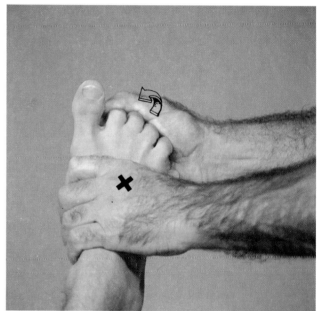

Fig. 127 a. Starting Position.

Procedure: Maintaining this grip, with the toes maximally flexed at the DIP and PIP joints, T then applies traction at the MTP joints while simultaneously *dorsal flexing* at the MTP joints and drawing the four toes towards the tibia.

Stimulation of Antagonists: T retains grip. T then asks P to move further in the direction of stretching, and resists that movement to stimulate P's antagonists.

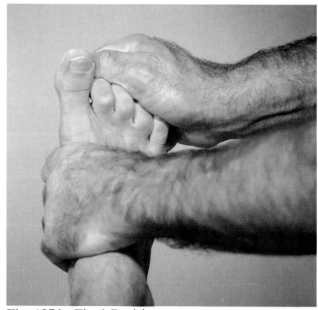

Fig. 127 b. Final Position.

PART 4

TABLES AND INDEX

The following tables list the various movements which may be restricted, indexed to the muscles which, when shortened, cause the restrictions.

The tables may be used diagnostically, to identify the muscles which may be involved in restricting particular movement. Or they may be used analytically, to identify the movements which may be restricted by the shortening of particular muscles.

In most, but not all cases, a shortened muscle causes restriction to motion in an opposite manner to its main action: a shortened extensor will restrict flexion; a shortened adductor will restrict abduction, and so on. In some cases actions and/or restricting effects may change when muscles are in extreme positions. For instance, most of the adductors of the hip can restrict extension when the hip is extended, but they also can restrict flexion when the hip is flexed.

The actions of many muscles effect more than one movement, frequently at more than one joint. Therefore, when one of these muscles is shortened, the restriction it causes at a joint often depends on the position of other joints at which it acts. For instance, the flexor digitorum superficialis of the forearm acts to flex the fingers, including at the PIP joints, volar flexes at the wrist, and flexes at the elbow. So the restrictions it may cause when shortened depend on an inter-relationship of these actions. It may:

– restrict extension and supination of the elbow and forearm when the fingers are extended,

– restrict dorsal flexion at the wrist when the fingers are extended,

– restrict extension at the MCP joints when the PIP joints are extended,

– restrict extension of the IP joints when the wrist is dorsally flexed, the elbow is extended, and the forearm is supinated.

Conditions for limited restriction, such as these for the flexor digitorum superficialis, are listed in the last column to the right in the tables involved. When the conditions listed are not fulfilled, the muscle involved may be considered not to restrict. For instance, when the fingers are flexed, a shortened flexor digitorum superficialis will not restrict dorsal flexion at the wrist (Table 4.4).

10.1. Table of
SHOULDER AND ARM MOVEMENTS RESTRICTED BY SHORTENED MUSCLES

●● = Primary restrictor   ● = Secondary restrictor

RESTRICTED MOVEMENT

SHORTENED MUSCLE	Flexion	Extension	Adduction	Abduction	Medial rotation	Lateral rotation
pectoralis major -abdominal part -clavicular part -sternocostal part	●● ●●	 ●●		●● ● ●●		● ● ●
latissimus dorsi	●●			●●		●
teres major	●●			●●		●●
biceps brachii -long head		●	●			●
deltoid -clavicular part -acromial part -spinal part	 ●	●●	 ●●	● ●	 ●	●
teres minor	●			●	●●	
infraspinatus	●				●●	
triceps brachii, -long head	●			●		
supraspinatus			●●		●	●
coracobrachialis	●	●		●		●
subscapularis	●			●		●●
biceps brachii -short head		●		●		●
pectoralis minor	●			(●)		(●)
subclavius	●			●		

165

SCAPULA AND CLAVICLE MOVEMENTS RESTRICTED BY SHORTENED MUSCLES

●● = Primary restrictor   ● = Secondary restrictor

RESTRICTED MOVEMENT

SHORTENED MUSCLE	Elevation	Depression	Adduction	Abduction	Medial rotation	Lateral rotation
subclavius	●●					
pectoralis minor	●●		●●			●●
serratus anterior	●		●●		●●	
trapezius -descending part -transverse part -ascending part	 ●●	 ●● ●		 ● ●● ●	 ●● ●●	
levator scapulae		●●		●		●
rhomboidei		●●		●●		●●
latissimus dorsi	●			●		
pectoralis major	●		●			

10.3. Table of
ELBOW AND FOREARM MOVEMENTS RESTRICTED BY SHORTENED MUSCLES

●● = Primary restrictor   ● = Secondary restrictor

RESTRICTED MOVEMENT

SHORTENED MUSCLE	Flexion	Extension	Pronation	Supination	Notes
biceps brachii -long head		●●	●		
-short head		●●	●		
brachialis		●●			
brachioradialis		●●	●	●	
pronator teres		●		●	
pronator quadratus				●	
triceps brachii	●●				
anconeus	●				
supinator		●	●●		
flexor carpi radialis		●		●	
flexor carpi ulnaris		●		●	
palmaris longus		●		●	
extensor carpi radialis longus		●	●		
extensor carpi radialis brevis		●	●		
extensor carpi ulnaris		●	●		
flexor digitorum superficialis		●		●	fingers extended
extensor digitorum communis		●	●		fingers flexed
extensor digiti minimi		●			finger flexed
extensor pollicis longus			●		thumb flexed
abductor pollicis longus			●		thumb adducted
extensor indicis			●		finger flexed
flexor pollicis longus		(●)	●	●	thumb extended

167

10.4. Table of
WRIST MOVEMENTS RESTRICTED BY SHORTENED MUSCLES

•• = Primary restrictor   • = Secondary restrictor

RESTRICTED MOVEMENT

SHORTENED MUSCLE	Volar flexion	Dorsal flexion	Radial flexion	Ulnar flexion	Notes
flexor carpi radialis		••		••	
flexor carpi ulnaris		••	••		
palmaris longus		•			
extensor carpi radialis longus	••			••	
extensor carpi radialis brevis	••				
extensor carpi ulnaris	••		••		
flexor digitorum profundus		•			finger extended
flexor digitorum superficialis		•			finger extended
extensor digitorum communis	••				finger flexed
extensor indicis	•			•	finger flexed
extensor digiti minimi	•				finger flexed
extensor pollicis longus	•			•	thumb flexed
extensor pollicis brevis	•			•	thumb flexed
abductor pollicis longus		•		•	adducted thumb
flexor pollicis longus		•			flexed thumb

10.5. Table of
METACARPO-PHALANGEAL (MCP) JOINT MOVEMENTS RESTRICTED BY SHORTENED MUSCLES

●● = Primary restrictor   ● = Secondary restrictor

RESTRICTED MOVEMENTS

SHORTENED MUSCLE	Flex-ion	Exten-sion	Abduc-tion	Adduc-tion	Opposi-tion	Reposi-tion	Notes
flexor digitorum profundus		●●					IP joint extended
flexor digitorum superficialis		●●					PIP joints extended
extensor digitorum communis	●●						DIP & PIP joints flexed
extensor indicis	●●						DIP & PIP joints flexed
extensor digiti minimi	●●						DIP & PIP joints flexed
lumbricales III-IV, I-II		●●					dorsal flexed wrist & flexed DIP & PIP joints
interossei dorsales I and II		●		●●			DIP & PIP joints flexed
interossei dorsales III & IV		●		●●			DIP & PIP joints flexed
interosseus palmaris I		●	●				DIP & PIP joints flexed
interossei palmaris II-III		●	●●				DIP & PIP joints flexed
abductor digiti minimi		●		●●	(●)		
flexor digiti minimi brevis		●●				●	wrist volar flexed; DIP & PIP joints flexed
opponens digiti minimi						●●	
extensor pollicis longus	●●				●●		wrist volar and ulnar flexed; IP joint flexed
extensor pollicis brevis	●●				●●		mainly with forearm pronated, & wrist ulnar flexed
flexor pollicis longus		●●				●●	mainly with wrist dorsal flexed & IP joint extended
flexor pollicis brevis		●●				●●	mainly with wrist dorsal flexed

FINGER (IP JOINT) MOVEMENTS RESTRICTED BY SHORTENED MUSCLES

●● = Primary restrictor   ● = Secondary restrictor

RESTRICTED MOVEMENT

SHORTENED MUSCLE	Flexion	Extension	Notes
flexor digitorum profundus		●●	mainly with wrist dorsal flexed & forearm supinated
flexor digitorum superficialis		●●	mainly with wrist dorsal flexed, elbow extended, and forearm supinated
extensor digitorum communis	●●		mainly with wrist volar flexed, elbow extended, and forearm pronated
extensor indicis	●●		mainly with wrist volar flexed, elbow extended, and forearm pronated
extensor digiti minimi	●●		mainly with wrist volar flexed, elbow extended, and forearm pronated
lumbricales	●●		mainly with wrist dorsal flexed and MCP joints extended
interossei dorsales I and II	●		mainly with MCP joints extended
interossei dorsales III-IV	●		mainly with MCP joints extended
interosseus palmaris I	●		mainly with MCP joints extended
interossei palmares II-III	●		mainly with MCP-joints extended
extensor pollicis longus	●●		mainly with forearm pronated, wrist volar & ulnar flexed, MCP joint flexed, and thumb opposed
flexor pollicis longus		●●	mainly with forearm supinated, wrist dorsal flexed, MCP joint extended, and thumb repositioned

10.7. Table of
MOVEMENTS OF THE CARPO-METACARPAL (CMC) JOINTS OF THE THUMB AND THE LITTLE FINGER RESTRICTED BY SHORTENED MUSCLES

●● = Primary restrictor   ● = Secondary restrictor

RESTRICTED MOVEMENT

SHORTENED MUSCLE	Flexion	Extension	Abduction	Adduction	Opposition	Reposition
extensor pollicis longus	●●				●	
extensor pollicis brevis	●●			(●●)	●	
abductor pollicis longus				●●	●	(especially with wrist ulnar & dorsal flexed)
flexor pollicis longus		●●				●●
flexor pollicis brevis		●●		●		●
opponens pollicis		●	●			●●
abductor pollicis brevis		●		●●		●
adductor pollicis		●	●●			●●
extensor digiti minimi	●●				●	
abductor digiti minimi		●		●●	●●	
flexor digiti minimi brevis		●●		●		
interosseus palmaris I		●	●●			

10.8. Table of
HIP MOVEMENTS RESTRICTED BY SHORTENED MUSCLES

●● = Primary restrictor   ● = Secondary restrictor

RESTRICTED MOVEMENT

SHORTENED MUSCLE	Flex-ion	Exten-sion	Abduc-tion	Adduc-tion	Medial rotation	Lateral rotation	Notes
iliopsoas		●●			●		
sartorius		●		●	●		
rectus femoris		●●					
pectineus		●●	●●		●		
tensor fasciae latae		●		●		●●	
gluteus maximus	●●		●	●	●●		
gluteus medius	●	●		●●	●●	●	
gluteus minimus	●	●		●●	●	●●	
biceps femoris -long head	●●		●		●		mainly with knee extended
semitendinosus	●●		●			●	mainly with knee extended
semimembranosus	●●		●			●	mainly with knee extended
gracilis		●	●●			●	mainly with knee extended
adductor longus		●	●●		●		
adductor brevis		●	●●		●		
adductor magnus	●	●	●●		●	●●	
piriformis	●			●	●●		
quadratus femoris	●		●		●●		
gemelli	●				●●		
obturator externus			●		●●		
obturator internus	●				●●		

10.9. Table of
KNEE MOVEMENTS RESTRICTED BY SHORTENED MUSCLES

●● = Primary restrictor   ● = Secondary restrictor

RESTRICTED MOVEMENT

SHORTENED MUSCLE	Flexion	Extension	Medial rotation	Lateral rotation	Notes
semitendinosus		●●		●(●)	mainly with hip flexed
semimembranosus		●●		●	mainly with hip flexed
biceps femoris		●●	●●		mainly with hip flexed
rectus femoris	●●				mainly with hip extended
vastus lateralis	●●		●		
vastus intermedius	●●				
vastus medialis	●●		(●)	(●)	
sartorius		●		●	mainly with hip extended
popliteus		●		●●	
gastrocnemius		●			
plantaris		●			
tensor fasciae latae	●		●		
gracilis		●		●	mainly with hip extended

10.10. Table of
ANKLE MOVEMENTS RESTRICTED BY SHORTENED MUSCLES

●● = Primary restrictor   ● = Secondary restrictor

RESTRICTED MOVEMENT

SHORTENED MUSCLE	Plantar flexion	Dorsal flexion	Inversion (supination)	Eversion (pronation)	Notes
tibialis anterior	●●			●●	
extensor digi- torum longus	●●		●●		
peroneus tertius	●●		●●		
extensor hallucis longus	●			●	mainly with great toe MTP & IP joints flexed
gastrocnemius		●●			mainly with knee extended
plantaris		●		●	mainly with knee extended
soleus		●●			
peroneus longus		●	●●		
flexor digitorum longus		●		●	mainly with MTP, PIP, and DIP joints extended
flexor hallucis longus		●		●	mainly with MTP & IP joints extended
tibialis posterior		●		●	
peroneus brevis		●	●●		

10.11. Table of
TOE MOVEMENTS RESTRICTED BY SHORTENED MUSCLES

●● = Primary restrictor ● = Secondary restrictor

RESTRICTED MOVEMENT

SHORTENED MUSCLE	Flexion	Extension	Abduction	Adduction	Notes
extensor digitorum longus	●●				mainly with ankle plantar flexed
extensor hallucis longus	●●				mainly with ankle plantar flexed
flexor digitorum longus		●●			mainly with ankle dorsal flexed
flexor hallucis longus		●●			mainly with ankle dorsal flexed
abductor hallucis				●●	
flexor digitorum brevis		●●			
abductor digiti minimi				●●	
quadratus plantae		●●			
lumbricales	●● DIP PIP	● MTP			mainly with ankle dorsal flexed and MTP joints extended
flexor hallucis brevis		●● MTP			
adductor hallucis		●	●●		
flexor digiti minimi brevis		●●		●	
interosseus dorsalis I	● IP	● MTP		●	mainly with MTP joints extended
interossei dorsales II-IV	● DIP PIP	● MTP	●		mainly with MTP joints extended
interossei plantares	● DIP PIP	● MTP	●		mainly with MTP joints extended
extensor digitorum brevis	●●				
extensor hallucis brevis	●● MTP		●		

INDEX OF MUSCLES